MAN IN COMMAND

HOW TO GO FROM THE MOST SELF-DOUBTING GUY IN THE ROOM TO THE MOST CONFIDENT MAN

DAVE BOWDEN

IRREVERENT GENT

Copyright © 2017 by Dave Bowden

All rights reserved.

No part of this book may be reproduced in any form or by any electronic or mechanical means, including information storage and retrieval systems, without written permission from the author, except for the use of brief quotations in a book review.

Disclaimer

The material in this book is for informational and entertainment purposes only. The author and publisher expressly disclaim responsibility for any adverse effects resulting from the use or application of the information contained in this book.

I, the author, hold no degrees in medicine, psychology, exercise physiology or style(ology?), nor am I an expert in any of those fields. (I do, however, have degrees in philosophy and journalism, so I *am* an expert at not getting a job after graduating.)

For Michelle.
Nothing gives me feel more in command,
or gives me as much confidence, as your love.

YOUR FREE GIFT

You're about to learn a comprehensive long-term strategy for becoming a strong, charming, self-confident man.

Developing real, deep, authentic self-confidence takes sustained time and effort – an effort that becomes a hell of a lot easier when you develop the right habits.

That's why, as a companion to *Man in Command*, I've put together a free e-book called *Highly Confident Habits: 22 Proven Ways to Think, Look and Feel Formidable.*

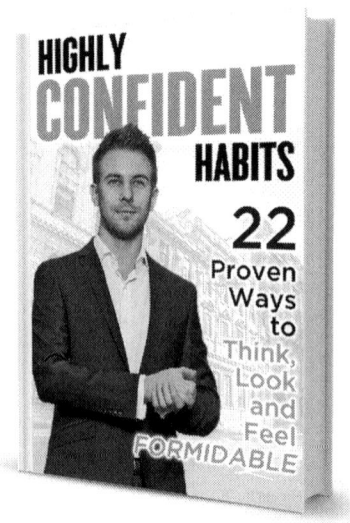

In this e-book you'll discover some quick and easy things you can do throughout the day – from the moment you wake up in the morning to right before you go to bed – to make yourself feel more calm, comfortable, charismatic and in control.

Check out www.IrreverentGent.com/Highly-Confident-Habits to claim your free copy.

INTRODUCTION

Reading the email, my hands start to shake and I feel a rumbling in the pit of my stomach. A familiar cocktail of nervousness, uncertainty and anxiety wells up inside me.

The magazine publishing company where I work has just posted an ad for my dream job, and I feel myself desperately wanting it and, simultaneously, completely fearing what I would do if I actually got it.

The company publishes fitness and health magazines, and I've spent the better part of the past three years as the managing editor of its two most successful titles – one dedicated to women's fitness and the other to healthy cooking. They're great magazines, but as neither a woman nor a cook, not especially applicable to my life.

Now, the top job at our fledgling brother publication, a men's fitness title meant to compete with industry heavyweights like *Men's Health* and *Men's Fitness*, has become available.

This is the opportunity every editor dreams of; it is the chance to move out of middle management and into the role of editor in chief, where I could actually help shape a magazine's editorial direction instead of just following marching orders.

As I skim through the job posting, I can't help but think that I'm actually pretty qualified for the role.

I have experience in almost every aspect of magazine publishing and have developed a solid reputation among my colleagues and senior management.

I'm a gym rat with years of firsthand experience navigating the ups and downs of the fitness lifestyle, and I can easily relate to the magazine's target reader.

And as second-in-command of the company's two most successful titles, I have plenty of experience dealing with the writers, editors, graphic designers, advertising department and every other position responsible for getting a magazine to press each month.

But just as my excitement begins to peak, almost as if on cue, it transforms into anxiety, dread and, inevitably, the desperate dance of excuse-making at which I'm all too skilled:

> "I mean, taking the reins of an entire magazine's editorial direction is a huge responsibility – I can't possibly be ready for that."

> "I may be a decent second-in-command, but being the top dog must require all sorts of intangible skills that I probably can't even fathom."

> "Plus, the job posting clearly says they want a minimum of five years of editorial management experience, and I only have three, so I'm actually not qualified at all."

> "OK, that seals it, I shouldn't even bother applying..."

And I didn't.

I didn't go to my boss, with whom I had a good relationship and who also happened to be in charge of hiring for this position, to tell him that I was interested.

I didn't ask any of my friends or colleagues about the pros and cons of applying.

I didn't start working on my resume or compiling writing samples.

In fact, I didn't say or do anything that would suggest I wanted the job.

And a few weeks later, the company announced that they had made an outside hire. Unlike me, he didn't actually have *any* editorial management experience, but he had a bunch of other advantages, so they felt like he'd be a good fit.

And just like that, my dream job was gone.

A Longtime Lack of Confidence

I wish I could tell you that I invented the anecdote above just for the sake of opening this book with a compelling little yarn.

Unfortunately, when it comes to stories about lacking self-confidence, I don't need to invent anything – I have a deep well of moments to draw from. Since you're reading this, you probably know these moments, too; they're the ones that make you feel like an insufficient, insecure impostor.

For the better part of a decade, from my late teens to my late twenties, I wasn't so much a "go-getter" as I was a "come-hither" (and yes, I'm fully aware of how creepy that sounds). I didn't take advantage of opportunities or make things happen. Instead I hesitated, worried, overthought to the point of inaction, and then regretted.

Again and again. And again.

In hindsight, it started in university, where I didn't have enough self-esteem to take even the most mundane of risks.

I didn't step foot in the gym during my freshman year because I was too intimidated and frightened by the prospect of looking like I didn't belong there.

I didn't ask out any girls because I was terrified of rejection.

I didn't apply for any on-campus jobs because I assumed I wasn't qualified.

I didn't join any clubs, enrol in any extracurriculars, apply to study abroad…

In short, I didn't take command of my life. In fact, I didn't do anything at all if it would have required me to "put myself out there."

And as if all of that passivity didn't sink my self-esteem enough, I'd dig the hole deeper by chastising myself for my lack of action. I used to trap myself in a negative feedback loop where I would:

1. Fail to take action and watch opportunities pass me by
2. Shit on myself for doing so
3. Feel even more worthless as a result of my own negative self-talk
4. Be even less likely to take action the next time – thus repeating the cycle

Sound familiar?

Recognizing Rock Bottom

This penchant for inaction and self-punishment continued well into my twenties; technically I was becoming a "man," but in my heart of hearts I still felt like the same nervous kid who waited too long to ask the girl he liked to prom, only to let another guy swoop in and ask her first. (Like I said – I've got *a lot* of stories like that.)

When I was younger, I used to think that these feelings of insecurity and inadequacy would somehow just dissipate when I "grew up," without my having to actually *do* anything.

But as I grew into a twenty-something man with the inner life of a scared teenager, I was forced to take a deep, honest look at myself and admit that if self-esteem hadn't somehow magically arrived yet, it probably wasn't coming.

Somewhere in my mid twenties, around the time I let my dream job slip away without making so much as a peep, I came to the realization that I actually had only two options:

1. I could do nothing – which is to say, continue what I had been doing – and live the rest of my days frequently feeling timid, nervous, resentful and full of regrets. Or,
2. I could do something, *anything* – exactly what, I didn't yet know – to bolster myself and finally take command of my life.

Putting it in such stark terms made the choice obvious.

I finally admitted to myself that if I was ever going to take command of my confidence – to overcome my overthinking and self-doubt, increase my levels of social comfort and charisma, and build the kind of self-esteem I needed to achieve my goals – I was going to have to get off my ass and start taking action.

Up until that point, I had spent twenty-odd years skimming the surface of life, and frequently found myself disappointed in the process.

It was finally time to dig in, and start laying a foundation for real, authentic, lasting self-confidence.

"Invest in Yourself"

I adopted "invest in yourself" as my simple (if a little clichéd) mantra and got *serious* about self-improvement.

I spent more than a decade reading, watching and listening to every piece of personal development advice I could get my hands on and learning as much as I could about how my mind works.

I spent countless days in the gym building a bigger, stronger body, and eventually discovered how good it feels to actually take pride in my physical presence.

I tried every conversation hack and socializing technique I could find, until I finally learned how to get over my nerves and confidently converse with anyone.

And I read fashion magazines, pored over menswear blogs and spent hours consulting with department store clerks to develop a sharp sense of personal style.

And somewhere along the way, something funny happened.

Forgetting Old Feelings

I originally started down the road of self-improvement because I felt insufficient in some vague but undeniable way. But as I focused on the areas of my life that I most wanted to improve, set goals for myself, and made progress on my objectives, I kind of – well, I don't know how else to put this – *forgot* about feeling insecure.

It's just hard to feel bad about yourself when you're making progress, week in and week out, on the goals you most want to achieve. Sure, I didn't transform from a snivelling geek to a swaggering superman overnight, like they often do in the movies. But eventually I really did get bigger, stronger, more confident and more self-reliant.

In short, I took command of my confidence. I didn't become arrogant, cocky, conceited or self-aggrandizing—at least, I certainly hope I didn't. (One of the many benefits of building hard-won, self-made self-confidence is that it also builds character, so when I finally achieved my goal and unleashed my inner lion, he was a lot more like Mufasa than Scar.)

By focusing on the pillars that were most important to me and working hard to methodically build up each one, I managed to take control of my life and create a solid, unshakeable foundation of confidence.

And you can too.

How to Become a Man in Command

This book is designed to help you strengthen your self-confidence in four fundamental domains:

- Your mindset
- Your body
- Your social skills
- Your style

The book is dedicated to helping you understand what confidence is, how it can fundamentally change the way you do everything – from getting out of bed in the morning to achieving your highest ambitions – and, most importantly, how you can acquire it.

Part 1: An Introduction to Self-Confidence

You probably already know that confidence is important (you wouldn't be reading this book if you didn't) but before you can solve a problem, you have to understand it. That's why chapter 1 breaks down the individual elements that contribute to self-confidence and gives you a better idea of why you feel the way you do about yourself.

With a definition of confidence established, in chapter 2 we'll explore what life looks like when you lack confidence. One word of warning: you're going to be tempted to skip this chapter. (I know, because I was tempted to not write it.) But don't skip it. Reminding yourself of how dire the consequences are when you lack confidence will provide the motivation you need to start building it.

Then in chapter 3, we'll review the other side of the coin – and inject a shot of positive motivation – by reviewing some of the (many!) advantages of increased confidence and self-esteem.

Once we've established what confidence is and why it's so important, it'll be time to get down to brass tacks. In parts 2, 3 and 4 you'll learn how to go from shy, quiet and self-doubting to strong, charming and self-confident.

Part 2: Cultivating a Confident Mindset

We'll start by focusing on your mindset. In chapters 4, 5 and 6 you'll learn techniques that have been proven to increase your levels of happiness, productivity and self-control, all of which lead to a greater command of your mental wellbeing, more contentment and more confidence. You'll also learn how to develop the healthy habits you need to continually feed your brain and expand your knowledge base perpetually.

Part 3: Build a Better Body, Build a Better You

After learning how to bolster your brain, we'll explore ways you can build your body. Chapters 7, 8 and 9 will focus on the three cornerstones of physical fitness: exercise, nutrition and sleep. Here you'll learn how to start – and, crucially, *stick to* – a workout plan, how to fuel your training and empower your body with clean, healthy foods, and how to make sure you're utilizing the body's secret weapon (spoiler alert: it's sleep) to its full restorative advantage.

Part 4: Solidify Your Social Skills

With your mind and body on the path to improved self-confidence, we'll shift our focus away from you and on to other people. In chapter 10 you'll learn a step-by-step method designed to help even the shyest of guys slowly, but surely, come out of their shells. In chapter 11 I'll share a dozen insightful socializing tips that will help you build on your momentum. Then in chapter 12, you'll discover a quick and deceptively effective trick you can use to turn anyone into a fast friend.

Part 5: Strengthen Your Style

After learning how to take command of your internal confidence by strengthening your mind, body and social skills, we'll take a look at ways you can project that confidence externally, by cultivating a look that's sharp and self-empowering. You'll learn how and why style strengthens your self-confidence, then you'll discover a proven method for not just looking more confident, but feeling it every time you get dressed. And to finish it off, I'll show you more than a dozen handsome hacks you can use to further refine your style and take your look to the next level.

By using the methods outlined above, I've managed to take command of my confidence and go from a shy, self-doubting guy who couldn't even work up the nerve to apply for a job he was qualified for to a strong, self-assured man who knows he's not just worthy, but capable of achieving anything he puts his mind to.

If my experience has taught me anything, it's this:

Self-confidence isn't something you're born with – it's something you build.

Head to chapter 1 now to start building yours.

PART I

WHAT CONFIDENCE IS, AND WHY YOU NEED IT

This book starts where any instructive text worth its salt should: at the end.

As Stephen Covey, author of the hugely influential *The 7 Habits of Highly Effective People*, wrote:

> "To begin with the end in mind means to start with a clear understanding of your destination. It means to know where you're going so that you better understand where you are now and so that the steps you take are always in the right direction." [1]

So before we deep dive into an exploration of *how* to take command of your confidence, let's start by exploring *what* confidence is and understanding how psychologists define it.

With the definition established and your goal clearly in mind, we'll then make sure you remain motivated to take the actions prescribed throughout the rest of the book, first by looking at the consequences of lacking confidence, and then by exploring the myriad ways confidence can change your life.

1
WHAT IS SELF-CONFIDENCE?

"Self-esteem is the disposition to experience oneself as being competent to cope with the basic challenges of life and of being worthy of happiness."

– Nathaniel Branden

As the old saying goes, if you don't know where you're going, you'll never get there. In my early twenties, when I was too afraid to put myself out there and try new things, I had an unmistakable sense that I wanted to change myself and improve, but I couldn't quite put my finger on how I wanted to change or who, exactly, I wanted to become.

To help you avoid making the same mistake and give you the clarity of purpose that I lacked, in this chapter we're going to define self-confidence in specific terms that will help you create a clear, focused picture of the man you want to be and what you want to achieve.

But before we dig into exactly what self-confidence is, let's take a second to clarify some terminology.

Self-esteem refers to how you feel about yourself overall. A person can have high self-esteem but find themselves feeling unconfident at certain tasks; for instance, after a lifetime spent studying and working in literary fields, I'm not at all confident in my ability to do math on the fly (a fact that can be corroborated by every restaurant server I've ever had, each of whom had to wait *very* patiently for me to calculate their tip).

But because I have high overall self-esteem, lacking confidence in certain areas where I know I'm low-skilled does not dramatically affect my overall sense of value or self-worth.

So, self-esteem is general, broad, and high-level; it refers to how you feel overall. Confidence, by contrast, is specific; it refers to how you feel about yourself in relation to distinct tasks or aspects of life.

In this chapter we'll use "confidence" to refer to two specific components of overall self-esteem, which I'll outline below. But since "self-esteem" is kind of a mouthful, throughout the rest of the book I'll just use the word "confidence" as a shorthand for the sort of deeply rooted, unshakeable, overall self-esteem you want to develop.

The Definition of Self-Esteem

One of the most comprehensive definitions of self-esteem was established by the psychotherapist and writer Nathaniel Branden. In his books *The Psychology of Self-Esteem* and *The Six Pillars of Self-Esteem*, Branden outlined a definition of self-esteem that consists of two main elements: self-efficacy and self-respect.

"Self-esteem, fully realized, is the experience that we are appropriate to life and to the requirements of life," Branden writes.

What does it mean to feel like you're "appropriate to life"? Branden argued that it consisted of confidence in two areas. First of all, confidence in our ability to cope with the basic challenges of life, and secondly, "confidence in our right to be successful and happy... entitled to assert our needs and wants, achieve our values and enjoy the fruits of our efforts."

Confidence in our ability to think and cope with life's challenges is what he called self-efficacy, while self-respect consists of confidence in our right to feel worthy.[2]

Unpacking Self-Esteem: Self-Efficacy and Self-Respect

Learning that self-efficacy and self-respect are the two central components of self-esteem can certainly be enlightening, but they don't exactly provide an "aha!" moment. In fact, they bring up an obvious next question: "OK – so how do we build them?"

Fortunately, Branden unpacked each element further, providing clues for how we can bolster each one in the process.

Self-efficacy, he explained, "means confidence in the functioning of my mind, in my ability to think, understand, learn, choose and make decisions; confidence in my ability to understand the facts of reality that fall within the sphere of my interests and needs; self-trust; self-reliance."[3]

So building self-efficacy means building "confidence in the functioning of my mind." That's good news for us, because in the four decades since Branden first published *The Psychology of Self-Esteem*, a lot of research has been done, and techniques developed, that can help us improve our mind's functionality. We'll explore three of the most fundamental of those in part 2 of this book.

Meanwhile, self-respect, the second aspect of self-esteem, "means assurance of my value; an affirmative attitude toward my right to live and to be happy; comfort in appropriately asserting my thoughts, wants and needs; the feeling that joy and fulfillment are my natural birthright."

This aspect of self-esteem can't be built quickly. Instead, it follows naturally from consistently performing a series of confidence-boosting actions over time.

Consistency = Competence = Confidence

As Branden lays out, self-esteem comes from self-efficacy and self-respect. But that's a bit of a mouthful, and repeating the word "self" that many times feels a little redundant.

So I like to shorten the equation to the three C's and say that Confidence comes from Consistency and Competence. It's easy to see how competence leads to confidence – we feel good about ourselves when we know we're able to perform at a high level those tasks we value most. But competence can also take time to cultivate, because any goal worth pursuing is probably not one you can get good at overnight.

Fortunately, you can build confidence before you build competency. Your confidence increases every time you practice, work and improve at a specific task, even if you haven't quite mastered it. So consistency builds confidence – you feel good about yourself knowing that you're working toward your goals. Consistency also builds competence – when you consistently work toward your goals, you get a little better each day. And this combination, consistency and competence, creates a deeply rooted, unshakeable confidence.

Cultivating Confidence

Parts 2, 3 and 4 of this book will show you how to consistently work toward worthy goals and develop competence in four areas of life that are essential to the modern man: your mindset, body, social skills and style. Using the advice laid out in those parts, you'll increase your self-efficacy and build self-respect in the process.

But, what if you don't? What if you don't take action, invest in yourself and consistently build competence and confidence?

Well, it won't be pretty, as we're about to learn.

2

WHY LACKING CONFIDENCE IS CATASTROPHIC

"Nothing holds you back more than your own insecurities."

– Susan Gale

Remember the story I told you in the introduction, about how I didn't believe in myself enough to even apply for a job I was imminently qualified for? When you don't have confidence in yourself, your abilities and your right to feel happy and fulfilled, a similar pattern and failure to take action emerges in almost every aspect of your life.

People with little to no self-confidence take fewer risks and are often too afraid to "put themselves out there" or reveal much about their personalities to others. As a result, they miss out on opportunities to learn, grow and improve that are essential for personal development.

"They become anxious about taking risks, trying something new, or expressing their opinion, because they're afraid of failure or looking foolish," writes Darlene Lancer, a marriage and relationship therapist, in an article for psychology website PsychCentral.com.

"The false belief about unworthiness undermines self-esteem and security and has serious consequences in your life."[4]

In this chapter we're going to explore a few of the most common – and catastrophic – of those consequences. As I mentioned earlier, I highly recommend you resist the urge to skip this chapter. It may be a little hard to read, but in this case, a little fear is actually a good thing.

Recognizing the all-too-real consequences of lacking confidence will motivate you to take action and follow through on the self-improvement advice you'll find in later chapters of this book.

Love, Romance and Relationships (or a Lack Thereof)

Finding and forging a loving relationship is difficult. Finding and forging a loving relationship when you're so scared of rejection that you can't even bring yourself to go looking for a partner? Practically impossible.

Just as I hesitated to apply for that job even though I was actually qualified, often people who are good catches and have a lot to offer romantically can find themselves too terrified to join a dating site or go out to bars and social events in search of potential partners.

As clinical psychologist Dr. Suzanne Lachmann puts it, "Nothing interferes with the ability to have an authentic, reciprocal relationship like low self-esteem. If you can't believe you're good enough, how can you believe a loving partner could choose you?"[5]

As if spending your life without a loving relationship weren't a large enough risk, it gets worse. Even if you somehow manage to find yourself in a relationship without having actively sought one out, chances are dangerously high that it will actually be the wrong kind of relationship.

"Those who are convinced that they're bad can end up in relationships with people who are emotionally or physically abusive, which reinforces and worsens their low self-esteem," explains Lancer.[6]

In short, lacking self-confidence can make it nearly impossible to find a relationship – especially the *right* kind of relationship.

Fitness and Health

Self-respect is one of the key components to self-esteem and overall confidence, but without it, you'll find it almost impossible to summon the willpower necessary to make healthy choices.

You won't be motivated to eat right, work out, get enough rest or keep yourself healthy if you don't have, as Nathaniel Branden put it earlier, "an affirmative attitude toward [your] right to live and to be happy."

Having enough self-respect to prioritize your health is the first step toward actually becoming strong and healthy. But unfortunately, it's far from the last. Even if you're sufficiently motivated to keep yourself in good shape, you're going to need the other component of confidence – self-efficacy – in order to achieve your health and fitness goals.

It's hard to build a better body if you're so nervous about going to the gym that you can't step foot inside one, or so intimidated by the guys at the health food store that you can't bring yourself to ask about supplements, or so afraid of interacting with people that you refuse to hire a personal trainer, or... well, you get the idea.

Getting healthier has a wonderful way of making you feel not just physically better, but mentally and emotionally better, too. But in most cases, you're going to need at least a little confidence in order to get started.

Career and Professional Life

It may not seem fair, but it is a documented fact: people with little self-esteem also get little respect at work.

Citing a study from Newcastle University and the University of Exeter in the United Kingdom, _Healthy Living_ magazine reports that "people who are underconfident in their own abilities are viewed as less able by their colleagues."[7]

At first glance, this probably sounds like an unfair piling on. After all, just because someone doesn't feel great about themselves doesn't mean they're not worthy of respect.

But when you consider the consequences of low confidence on one's job performance, the lack of respect can seem much more justified. In *The Six Pillars of Self-Esteem*, Branden provides a hypothetical, but all-too relatable example:

> A man receives a promotion in his company and is swallowed by panic at the thought of not possibly being able to master the new challenges and responsibilities. "I'm an impostor! I don't belong here!" he tells himself. Feeling in advance that he is doomed, he is not motivated to give his best. Unconsciously he begins a process of self-sabotage: coming to meetings underprepared, being harsh with staff one minute and placating and solicitous the next, clowning at inappropriate moments, ignoring signals of dissatisfaction from his boss. Predictably, he is fired. "I knew it was too good to be true," he tells himself."[8]

Lacking confidence, then, can be a career killer not just because it causes your colleagues to disrespect you, but because it actually gives them a fair reason for doing so.

Exploring the Opposite

Clearly the cost of lacking confidence is high: from the office to the bar and nearly everywhere in between, every aspect of your life is negatively affected when you don't feel confident and self-assured.

But what does the opposite look like? What would your life look like if you could summon confidence in every area that's most important to you?

Let's find out.

3

THE (MANY) BENEFITS OF BEING CONFIDENT

"Self-confidence is the first requisite to great undertakings."

– Samuel Johnson

Before we go any further, I just want to pause and double check:

You read that last chapter, right? You didn't skip it because you thought that you, of all people, don't need to be reminded of the consequences of low confidence. You didn't start it and then skip ahead when it started sounding uncomfortably familiar, right?

Right?

OK, good. Because now that we've done the difficult and, admittedly, perhaps a bit painful work of establishing what's at stake, we can move on to the *much* more empowering task of considering what kind of outcomes are possible – and even probable – for you when you have confidence.

In order to get anywhere, you have to know where you're going. So to make sure you're properly motivated to take action, in this chapter we're going to explore the many benefits of putting in the legwork required to build real confidence.

The Broad Benefits of Being Confident

Imagine waking up in the morning and feeling so excited about the day ahead that you practically leap out of bed.

You're not *concerned* about the assignments or projects you have to do, you *look forward* to them, because you know you have the drive, determination, skills and competencies needed to tackle them, and you're excited about the rewards that will come as a result.

You're not dreading going to the gym or trying to rationalize your way out of going today; instead, you're looking forward to it because you set a personal best on the bench press two days ago and today you plan to surpass it.

You're not nervous about going out to the bar after work; you're looking forward to meeting up with friends at the end of the day. Plus, you're going to that bar with the cute bartender you've been flirting with for a month now, and you're ready to ask her out.

You open your dresser and grab one of your favorite, perfect-fitting V-neck sweaters – the ones that always make you look fit and strong. You look in the mirror and like what you see. You're ready.

Just as the rising tide lifts all boats, increasing your self-confidence makes pretty much every aspect of your day – and your life – better.

Confident people are quicker to take risks and more resilient in the face of failure, allowing them to learn from their mistakes and try again with a higher likelihood of success. This creates a positive feedback loop:

Try > Fail > Learn > Grow >
Try Again > Succeed(!) >
Try Again > Fail > Learn > Grow >
Try Again > Succeed Again(!)
Et cetera

Because confidence makes you more willing to "put yourself out there," new opportunities arise for you. These lead to yet more opportunities and experiences, expanding your horizon and increasing the breadth of your knowledge, social circles and spheres of influence.

And because they have an established record of risk-taking, confident people are able to live without regrets. You don't need to waste time wondering what might have been if you actually tried. If it didn't work, you only need to ask why, then iterate and try again.

Like we did in the last chapter, let's take a look at a few specific realms of life. But instead of outlining the consequences of low confidence in each area, let's examine what can happen when you're confident and self-assured.

Love, Romance and Relationships

It probably seems obvious, but it bears saying: when you have more confidence, you get more dates.

Building self-confidence will help you bolster your romantic life in multiple ways, and the first one owes to basic math: the more people you ask out, the more dates you'll go on. And the more confident you feel, the more likely you'll be to ask someone out.

But confidence won't just help you ask the question, it'll make you more likely to get the answer you want. In their book *Compelling People*, authors John Neffinger and Matthew Kohut explain that when we're sizing up another person, there are only two traits that we're looking for: strength and warmth.

"People who project both strength and warmth impress us as knowing what they are doing and having our best interests at heart, so we trust them and find them persuasive," they write.[9]

When you display confidence – say, by taking a risk, putting yourself out there and asking someone out – you inherently display strength, which immediately makes you more attractive to your potential date.

And even if your confidence doesn't convince her to go out with you, it will help you bounce back from the rejection and try again – and keep trying until you succeed.

Friendships and Socializing

Developing deeply rooted confidence won't just help your romantic prospects, it will bolster both the quantity and quality of your platonic relationships too.

People who have more uncertainty and anxiety than confidence and self-esteem tend to look inward and obsess over their own insecurities, worries and doubts. Confident people, by contrast, worry less about themselves and their positions in the world, freeing them up to take a more active interest in the lives of those around them.

By inquiring about people at school, work and in their extended social circles, confident people can't help but collect friends (or at the very least, friendly acquaintances).

While these relationships often start out as arms-length or informal friendships they can lead to deeper relationships over time. Asking seemingly innocuous questions such as "How are you today?" or "What did you get up to last night?" may seem superficial at first, but it opens the door to further discussion and potentially more revealing conversations, which help pave the way for deep, trust-based relationships.

Being able to both acquire and deepen relationships with relative ease has plenty of benefits, besides just giving you plenty of social options on a Saturday night. Because confident people have both a wide network of friends and deeper relationships with many of the people in their network, they're much less prone to feelings of loneliness or inadequacy.

In addition, having an expanded social circle also offers more opportunities in almost every realm of life, from romance to career advancement. The more people you know, the more likely you'll be to hear about a job opening that just became available, or a woman who just became single and might be a good match for you.

Fitness and Health

Confidence has a symbiotic relationship with fitness and health.

On the one hand, there are few feelings more confidence-boosting than the accomplishment and pride that comes from finishing a tough workout. On the other hand, the more you value yourself and your capabilities, the more motivated you'll be to keep yourself healthy and get to the gym in the first place.

While it may not be clear which one is the cause and which one the effect, it's abundantly clear that confidence and fitness go hand in hand. Exercise releases endorphins and other confidence-boosting chemicals that will not only make you feel good while you're working out, but keep you feeling good the rest of the day.

Of course, exercise and healthy eating will also help you look better, which further compounds your confidence and bolsters your self-esteem every time you look in the mirror – or better yet, catch someone staring admirably at the fit silhouette you're able to project.

Career and Professional Life

Confidence won't just improve your performance in the gym: it'll help you at the office too.

According to *Forbes*, 61 percent of employers rank confidence as the most important trait they look for when hiring new employees. Some even rank it even more highly than skills.[10]

And just as confident people not only make more friends but also build better, deeper relationships, in a professional context confidence won't just help you land a job, it will make you much more likely to advance.

"A study of more than 500 students, academics and workers, published in the *Journal of Personality and Social Psychology*, showed that those who appeared more confident achieved a higher social status than their peers," reports the UK's *Telegraph*.[11]

Surprisingly, this holds true even in cases in which confident people have fewer skills than their low-confidence colleagues. The magazine *Healthy Living*, reporting on another study out of the UK, found that when managers are assessing who's ready for promotion, confidence stood out far above other traits.[12]

Cultivating Concrete Confidence

From your love life and your career to your friendships and your waistline, we've seen how confidence has the power to transform almost every aspect of your life – so it's time to start building it.

The rest of this book will be dedicated to helping you cultivate deep, authentic, concrete confidence by showing you how to:

- Cultivate an abundant, optimistic and confident mindset
- Build a strong, healthy body you can be proud of
- Overcome social hang-ups and bolster your people skills and charisma, and
- Project poise and power by stepping up your style

To develop a confident mindset, you'll first need to learn how to silence self-doubt, quiet your inner critic and think more abundantly.

Turn the page to find out how to get started.

PART II

CULTIVATING A CONFIDENT MINDSET

To escape insecurity and start building self-confidence, you need to understand how your mind works, then learn how to orient it toward thoughts of optimism, possibility, positivity and success.

In this part, you'll learn three proven techniques that will help you do just that. In chapter 4 you'll discover an ancient (and science-backed) technique for understanding your mind and remaining calm and confident. In chapter 5 you'll learn how to start each day feeling more content with yourself and more optimistic about your potential. Then chapter 6 will show you how to train your brain to learn and grow perpetually.

4

MEDITATION: A (SURPRISINGLY EFFECTIVE) WAY TO GET CALM, COOL AND COLLECTED

"If you want to understand your mind, sit down and observe it."

– Anagarika Munindra,
Buddhist monk

To many of us, meditation invokes images of bald men sitting in Tibetan temples, wrapped in red linen robes and chanting lyrically to themselves.
"Ohmmmmmmmm."

There's no doubt that those guys seem pretty chill, but you could be forgiven for thinking that taking up a similar practice is unlikely to help you lose weight, get a promotion, land a date or achieve any of your other goals.

But don't let the dharma deter you: a significant (and continually growing) body of scientific evidence suggests that meditation can have a real, measurable and dramatic impact on your life and well-being – and that includes your confidence.

Increased Happiness

In a 2008 study published in the *Journal of Personality and Social Psychology*, researchers took a group of working adults and randomly assigned half the group the task of practicing a loving-kindness meditation, what Buddhists call a "metta" meditation.

"This meditation practice produced increases over time in daily experiences of positive emotions, which, in turn, produced increases in a wide range of personal resources," the study reported.[13]

Meditation led to a decrease in illness symptoms and bolstered personal resources like mindfulness and purpose in life. What's more, the incremental gains the meditators made in these areas led to increased life satisfaction overall and a reduction in depression over time.

The results of the study suggest that if you're looking to build self-confidence, setting aside a few minutes each day to increase your sense of purpose in life and decrease your levels of stress and illness is a pretty great place to start.

Improved Self-Control

How do you handle stress, setbacks or disappointments? Let me guess: you let them roll right off your back, barely registering it as a blip on the radar before graciously moving on to tackle your next challenge.

Yeah, me neither.

Instead, I'm much more likely to let the negative feedback gnaw at me. Depending on the circumstances, I may lash out at the people around me, or internalize it and spend the following days (or even weeks) obsessing over how it happened and rationalizing why it happened – often making excuses for myself in the process. Or at least, that's what I used to do.

Since I began a daily meditation practice, I've found it much easier to take things in stride, and resist the urge to fly off the handle when something doesn't go my way. And a 2013 study from Stanford Medicine may explain why.

Researchers split a group of people up into two camps: one was a control group, and the other was assigned nine weeks of meditation, or "compassion cultivation training," to use their jargon.

The Stanford study reaffirmed the results of previous meditation studies, finding that meditation "resulted in increased mindfulness and happiness," and emphasized a further benefit that helps explain why it helps me – and you, and anyone else who meditates – handle stress and setbacks with more aplomb. In addition to making us feel happier and less stressed, meditation makes us more psychologically "flexible and adaptive," which leads to "reductions in worry and emotional suppression," the study found.

Being able to handle life's ups and downs while remaining (relatively) calm, cool and collected is a sure sign of self-confidence. And meditation, as it turns out, is a free, easy and effective way to help you get there.

Improved Productivity

If sitting around and thinking about nothing doesn't exactly scream "productivity," to you, I don't blame you. But as it turns out, meditation is one of the best ways to get more done.

Studies of intensive meditation practices have shown that meditation increases your memory and helps you remain focused and on-task. "Meditative training can improve performance on a novel task that requires the trained attentional abilities," as one study published in the journal PLOS Biology put it.[14]

While that particular study examined the effects of intensive meditation, others have looked at whether or not brief meditation can have similarly positive benefits—and found good news for anyone whose calendar can't accommodate a month-long meditation retreat. "Brief meditation training reduced fatigue, anxiety, and increased mindfulness," according to researchers from Wake Forest University School of Medicine. "Moreover, brief mindfulness training significantly improved visuo-spatial processing, working memory, and executive functioning."

"[These] findings suggest that four days of meditation training can enhance the ability to sustain attention – benefits that have previously been reported with long-term meditators."[15]

So if sitting on your duff for half an hour doesn't sound like the best way to plough through your day's to-do list, think again.

Making an investment in meditation will pay huge dividends over the long term.

How Meditation Boosts Self-Confidence

Becoming happier, improving your self-control and increasing your productivity all sound like worthwhile endeavors. But let's get to the heart of it: how does all this mindfulness make you more confident?

If you'll recall from chapter 1, psychologist Nathaniel Branden defined self-esteem – a.k.a. confidence – as a mix of self-efficacy and self-respect. In his book *The Six Pillars of Self-Esteem* Branden goes on to explain the six elements that are essential for developing confidence.

He describes the first pillar – the most fundamental foundation of self-esteem – as the practice of living consciously. "To live consciously means to seek to be aware of everything that bears on our actions, purposes, values and goals – to the best of our ability, whatever that ability may be."

Meditation is the most effect way to increase your ability and improve your awareness of your thoughts and feelings. This increased awareness makes you better able to assess your self-efficacy accurately, which in turn affects your self-worth.

A Real-World Example

I play on a beer league softball team. If you were to rank each of my team members in terms of ability, I would fall squarely in the middle of the pack: I hit consistently, but not powerfully, I run decently, but not lights-out, and I have a pretty good glove, but I make my share of errors. In short, I'm a pretty average player.

But when I make an error that costs my team a run, I have an unhelpful tendency to get especially hard on myself: I chastise myself for dropping a ball I think I should have had and curse myself under my breath. In those moments I'm embarrassed, and I allow myself to believe that I'm not an average player who made a mistake, but a terrible player not capable of doing better. This attitude eats up my attention and poisons the rest of my game, throwing me off at the plate and making me nervous every time another ball gets hit my way.

Or at least, it did.

One fall, after the softball season ended in September, I started meditating regularly. The habit stuck, and became a daily practice (eventually – I'll explain how I did it below). And after six months of meditating every day, I was shocked at the difference it made when I took the field the following April.

I certainly wasn't any more proficient a player – in fact, I was another year older and slower. But my attitude – and more specifically my assessment of my own ability and my role on the team – was completely different. I dropped just as many balls as I had the previous season, but I didn't beat myself up about it. I shrugged it off, chocked it up to the fact that I don't play or practice all that often, and put it out of my mind.

As a result, I was not just a better player that season, but a better teammate. I had a more positive attitude during each game, and since I wasn't bogged down by deluded thoughts of my own deficiency, I was much more willing to let go of my mistakes, focus on the next play, cheer on my teammates and help them improve.

Meditating didn't help us win more games, but it helped me have a hell of a lot more fun.

How to Develop a Meditation Practice

Meditating proved to be beneficial for me, but that doesn't mean it was easy – at least not at first. I remember the first time I ever tried it.

I put a pillow on the floor and sat down with my legs crossed, my back straight, my shoulders pulled back and my hands resting gently on my knees. I closed my eyes, and breathed in slowly. To an outside observer, I no doubt would have looked like the very pinnacle of meditative calmness.

It felt completely ridiculous.

It wasn't until a few months later that I learned I wasn't alone in feeling funny during my first foray into meditation. The vast majority of first-time meditators initially feel uncomfortable or even intimidated by its very prospect – even those who know about its science-backed benefits.

Fortunately, meditation is just like anything else: it can be broken down into small steps, which can lead to big results over time. Follow the steps below to ease yourself into meditation and begin to rewire your brain for more self-confidence.

Step 1: Start Small

As studies have shown, you can reap huge rewards from just a small amount of meditation. In the early going, your goal is simply to develop the habit of meditation, not to meditate for any specific length of time.

To make it easy on yourself, shoot for just five minutes of meditation each day for the next two weeks. No matter how busy you are, everyone can spare a measly five minutes a day, especially for something with so many potential benefits.

Don't worry about what time of day you're meditating; I enjoy doing it as part of my morning routine, while others find it relaxing to do before bed. Just work it into your day wherever you can.

Step 2: Seek Guidance

Beginner meditators often find it helpful to be guided through the meditative process by someone more experienced, who can help you focus your mind and navigate its many potential distractions.

While previous generations of meditators had to traverse the globe and trek up mountains to seek this kind of precious guidance, you and I just need a phone and some decent Wi-Fi.

There's a growing number of free and paid mobile apps designed to help ease you into the meditative process, but one of my favorite resources is YouTube, where aspiring gurus have taken the time to record thousands of guided meditations.

Simply search for phrases like "five-minute mindfulness meditation" or "beginner meditation" to find clips that cater to beginners.

When I began meditating, my personal favorite was a ten-minute track by author and neuroscientist Sam Harris, who calmly and slowly lays out exactly what you should do, and helps you navigate some of the speed bumps that will inevitably come up in your mind.

Step 3: Call Yourself Out

When you first begin practicing mindfulness you may find it difficult to focus on your breath or the sensations in your body. You may enjoy a few moments with a mind as calm as water, but it won't be long before thoughts enter your mind and send ripples through your serenity, distracting you from your intended area of focus.

This is totally normal, and over time you'll find it easier to let thoughts move into and out of your mind quickly. But in the beginning, when you notice that your mind has wandered somewhere you didn't intend for it to go, you might find it helpful to explicitly acknowledge your wayward thoughts.

When you catch your mind wandering, try saying something to yourself, like "thinking" or "back to the breath," to return your focus to where it should be at that moment. When my mind wanders during meditation, I've found it helpful to mentally say "thinking" and then imagine my thought as a bright red balloon. The balloon and its associated thought then float effortlessly out of my mind, allowing me to return to a relaxed and focused state.

Step 4: Forgive Yourself

In the beginning, you may find yourself using this balloon technique often, frequently interrupting your meditation practice in order to release your thoughts from your mind. It's tempting to beat yourself up for all this disruptive thinking, but resist that urge.

Everyone struggles with releasing their thoughts at first. After all, for most of your life you've done just the opposite: when a thought – about what you have to do today, or how something or someone made you feel, or anything else for that matter – enters your mind, you routinely follow it, get caught up in it and allow it to affect your mood, your actions and your life.

The reason you're practicing mindfulness meditation is to reduce the effect your thoughts have on your mood and disposition, thus becoming more relaxed and confident – but this takes time.

Don't be discouraged if you feel like you're still "thinking too much" after just a few meditation sessions. Stay with it and stay diligent in acknowledging when you're thinking and releasing your thoughts.

You'll never completely stem the tide of thoughts running through your mind, but by developing the practice of acknowledging and releasing them, you can transform yourself into a much cooler, calmer and more confident person.

5
GRATITUDE = GREATNESS

"Reflect upon your present blessings, of which every man has plenty; not on your past misfortunes, of which all men have some."

– Charles Dickens

During periods of low self-esteem, we often fall victim to that oh-so-human temptation to focus on what we don't have – and ignore all that we do have.

Remember earlier when I mentioned my habit of shitting on myself during softball games whenever I would make a mistake? I would curse the fact that I wasn't a better hitter, a faster runner, a more dependable defender and a better player overall.

But in those moments of self-pity, I was completely ignoring the other side of the coin: what allowed me to play softball in the first place. The only reason I was out on that field was because I was healthy and able-bodied. I had friends who liked me enough to invite me onto their team. I was familiar with the game because my parents had enrolled me early in T-ball and then supported me as I grew up and moved to increasingly more difficult leagues.

A few mistakes notwithstanding, I had a lot going for me as both a player and a person – I just needed to find a way to see the forest for the trees.

You can probably relate to this feeling. In your quest to build self-confidence, at one time or another you may have found yourself wishing you had a better body, a more positive or assertive attitude, better social skills, more friends, better clothes, more money or any number of other attributes.

And because you're so focused on your perceived deficits, you're likely ignoring or taking for granted your many blessings, which include everything from physical necessities like the shelter and food that ensure your continued survival, to mental assets like your self-awareness and willingness to change. (After all, you picked up this book, didn't you?)

Confident people take the opposite approach. By focusing on – and frequently reminding themselves of – everything that they have, they develop the positivity, self-belief and optimism that propels them toward new and exciting challenges.

Because they're better at focusing on what they do have, confident people take more risks, are better able to put their failures in perspective, and bounce back from setbacks quicker and with greater ease, learning from their mistakes and course-correcting in order to do better next time. All of which offers a pretty good argument for going from a "have not" to a "have" attitude.

Fortunately, a large (and continually growing) body of scientific evidence suggests that identifying and focusing on what you're grateful for, no matter how small, can actually have a tremendous impact on your happiness, health and confidence.

In this chapter you'll learn about some of the (many!) benefits of practicing gratitude and discover a method for becoming more grateful – and more confident – in just five minutes a day.

The Confidence-Boosting Benefits of Gratitude

Scientists – most notably Robert Emmons, a psychologist at the University of California Berkeley and author of *Thanks! How the New Science of Gratitude Can Make You Happier* – have shown that practicing gratitude offers myriad psychological, emotional, social and even physical benefits.

Below you'll find a few of the benefits most relevant to increasing your self-confidence, but you can discover even more on the website for UC Berkeley's Greater Good Science Center or GGSC (ggsc.berkeley.edu).

Increased Happiness

It's hard to be confident without being content. When you can appreciate, and even revel in, all that you have in life, you exude a contentment and confidence that others find both attractive and inspiring.

Science has shown that by actively working to increase your level of gratitude, you can develop just such a mindset.

"Practicing gratitude has proven to be one of the most reliable methods for increasing happiness and life satisfaction," according to Berkeley's Greater Good Science Center. "It also boosts feelings of optimism, joy, pleasure, enthusiasm, and other positive emotions."[16]

Strengthened Relationships

In addition to providing the contentment and confidence to attract new friends and loved ones into your life, gratitude can help bolster relationships you may currently take for granted.

Many of us overlook and undervalue those who are closest to us. We erroneously assume that thanks to proximity or societal norms, our parents, siblings, friends and other close relations have to like us – not because we're worthy of their love, but because they feel a social obligation to do so.

But when you focus on gratitude, you start to see all the things your friends, family, colleagues and mentors do not because they have to, but because they want to.

In addition to the many kindnesses they pay you, the people in your life further enrich you simply by having rich lives of their own. They have character traits you can observe and emulate (or character flaws you can try to avoid); personal anecdotes you can learn from, even – and especially – if they differ from your own experience; and relationships with other people whom they can bring into your life, enriching you further.

In short, thinking gratefully means being more conscious of the people in your life, which makes you feel closer and more connected to them.

In short, gratitude "makes us feel closer and more committed to friends and romantic partners," according to the GGSC.

Improved Physical Health

This might be one of the most surprising and straight-up awesome benefits of gratitude. You would expect gratitude to have a positive effect on your mindset, but few people would suspect that increasing your level of gratefulness can also have such a positive effect on your body.

The connection between your mind and your body is a two-way street. Improve your body by exercising, eating well and getting enough rest, and you can improve your mind thanks to increased brain function and the release of happiness-inducing chemicals like dopamine. Conversely, when you focus on gratitude and take other steps to improve your mental health, your body will reap significant rewards.

"Gratitude strengthens the immune system, lowers blood pressure, reduces symptoms of illness, and makes us less bothered by aches and pains," reports the GGSC. "It also encourages us to exercise more and take better care of our health."

Increased Compassion

When you're more grateful for what you have, you're more likely to help those who have less. "Grateful people are more helpful, altruistic, and compassionate," says the GGSC.

Science has shown that increasing your level of compassion comes with myriad other benefits, including an increased motivation to take action, a reduced fear of suffering and greater calmness and ability to handle stressful situations, among other advantages.

How to Get More Grateful, Five Minutes at a Time

Self-confidence follows from taking positive action, and by now I hope you're convinced that there are few actions more positive and confidence-boosting than those that increase your level of gratitude.

But while we all intuitively understand what it's like to feel grateful, you're probably not used to thinking of gratitude as a practice, which leads us to ask: what can you do to feel more grateful?

Fortunately, science has the answer – and more fortunately still, all it requires is a pen or pencil, some paper, and a few minutes each day.

The GGSC recommends what it calls the "Three Good Things" exercise. At the end of the day, you simply write down three things that went well for you, along with a brief explanation of why they went well. Do this every day for at least a week.

Interestingly, it doesn't matter how big or small your three things are. They could be as miniscule as someone smiling at you, or as huge as landing your dream job or scoring a date with the girl of your dreams. The important thing is that you write them down, which helps anchor them in your mind.

And lest you think this little exercise sounds more like fluffy feel-goodery than cold hard science a study published in the journal *American Psychologist* backs it up.

The study's authors directed people to a website where they were instructed to write down three things they were grateful for each day.

The results? The exercise was associated with increased happiness, not just for the moments immediately following the writing, but for the following six months![17]

Try this exercise for yourself to start increasing your levels of health, happiness, gratitude and self-confidence.

I think you'll find that a few minutes each day is a small price to pay for six months of increased happiness and confidence.

6

THE READING HABIT

(This book's not bad – but it's not enough)

"A reader lives a thousand lives before he dies… The man who never reads lives only one."

– George R.R. Martin

Every aspect of life that's ever made me feel nervous, intimidated or downright scared was one I didn't really understand.

For instance, before I picked up a fitness magazine and started learning about exercise and nutrition science, the prospect of going to the gym horrified me.

And when I walked into a clothing store I wouldn't even want the sales staff to look at me, lest I betray the fact that I knew nothing about menswear – until I started reading *GQ* and stumbled upon the internet's abundance of men's fashion blogs.

Likewise, just thinking about making small talk with strangers at a party (or more terrifying still, with women at a bar!) was enough to cover me in a flop sweat, until I discovered that bookstores carry reams of titles about talking to people and improving your social skills.

It turns out G.I. Joe was right: knowing really is half the battle. In fact, he may have undersold the case.

As I started educating myself about the things that previously scared me the most, I came to realize that the only reason these topics had been so intimidating in the past was because I was so ignorant about them. By learning about them – hell, just by realizing that they could be learned – I demystified them.

In my mind, things like building muscle, developing social skills and becoming a well dressed man transformed from fantasies that eluded me to subjects I could study. And as a proud and self-proclaimed nerd, studying was one thing I knew I could do.

Just as I was more comfortable writing essays and taking tests after I had studied, I became more comfortable going to the gym, talking to strangers and dressing well once I had learned about the principles and strategies that underlie those (previously sweat-inducing) endeavors.

You can develop the same comfort and confidence in the areas that interest you most by developing a simple habit: reading.

Every. Damn. Day.

How to Develop the Reading Habit

Reading how-to guides about subjects you're interested in may not sound like particularly complicated advice (after all, you're doing it right now!), but be honest with yourself: how often do you actually finish the books that you read?

If you're anything like me, the answer is never, but you tell people it's "not as often as I'd like." Many a third act and final chapter has gone directly from my nightstand to my bookshelf without so much as a glance, despite my enthusiasm when I first bought the book.

It wasn't until I succeeded in turning reading into an automatic part of my day that I (finally) started finishing books with any regularity. In doing so, I dramatically increased my understanding of topics as varied as conversation skills, psychology, leadership, personal finance and investing, and significantly boosted my self-confidence in the process.

Follow the steps below to take reading from a "have to" to a habit, and you'll be richly rewarded (especially if you make it all the way to the final chapter of this book, which has some excellent advice about how to look your best).

Step 1: Pick a Time, Any Time

The first key to making reading a habit is to choose a time of day when you can, will and – crucially – will *want* to do it every day. Ask yourself: are you a morning person or a night owl?

Do you already have a morning or evening routine into which you could easily slot a few minutes for reading?

Think carefully about your daily schedule and pre-existing habits and schedule some reading time for wherever it seems most natural.

Step 2: Set a Limit, Read Within It

If you perceive reading as something that requires a large commitment of either time or mental energy, it will quickly come to feel like a monotonous chore rather than a valuable confidence-booster.

To keep this from happening, make sure you set either a time or page limit each day, and then stick to it. For instance, commit to reading just ten pages of a good book each day, even if you find you're flying through those pages quickly or stopping before you can really get into a good flow state.

The goal is to train your brain to think of your daily reading habit as something so short and easy that you'd feel silly not doing it. This tactic has the added benefit of leaving you wanting more, which will make you not just likely, but even hungry to pick up where you left off tomorrow.

Step 3: Go from Page to Practice

Finally, if you're reading a book that offers advice about a subject or skill you're trying to learn, put that advice to work right away.

Trying what the book recommends will either affirm that the advice is sound, and encourage you to keep reading and progressing through its recommended steps, or reveal that it's nonsense and allow you to put the book down and stop wasting your time on it.

You can start by performing a (ridiculously meta) test of these very steps. If you've been struggling to read or return to this book on a regular basis, try implementing the reading habit over the next week.

Best case scenario? It will work, and you'll soon know exactly how to take control of your confidence.

Worst case? Well, at least you won't have to put up with any more of my lame jokes.

PART III

BUILD A BETTER BODY, BUILD A BETTER YOU

When it comes to building self-confidence, your body is an obvious – and fundamental – place to focus, because it underlies so much of what makes you... well, you.

Improving both your body and your perception of that body will have trickle down effects that will bolster your confidence in each of the other areas mentioned in this book: your mindset, your social skills and your style.

In this part you'll learn how to improve the three most important elements of your physical health – fitness, nutrition and recuperation – by discovering a proven process for starting a workout plan and motivating yourself to keep at it consistently; learning how to accelerate your efforts by cleaning up your diet; and finding out how to improve both the quality and quantity of your sleep – and why it's so damn important.

7
STARTING – AND STICKING TO – A WORKOUT PLAN

"Physical fitness is not only one of the most important keys to a healthy body, it is the basis of dynamic and creative intellectual activity."

– John F. Kennedy

Building a body you can be proud of doesn't mean you have to pack on muscle like Dwayne "The Rock" Johnson, or trim yourself down to 10 percent body fat like Zac "High School Musical" Efron. (Yeah, I'm not thrilled with the *High School Musical* reference either, but I'll be damned if the guy ain't ripped.)

But it does mean you have to keep yourself feeling strong, healthy and fit, which is going to require a regular workout plan, no matter what body type you're striving toward.

And as anyone who's ever made a New Year's resolution knows, starting a workout plan is tough. And sticking to it? That's Navy SEAL tough.

But it really doesn't have to be.

In this chapter you'll learn a straightforward, step-by-step process you can use to get motivated, start a workout plan, tailor it to your schedule and (this part is key) keep at it week after week.

Step 1: Choose a Body Avatar

If you want to not only start working out but keep working out until you get your desired result, you have to define what that result is. The best way to do this is to create a vivid and detailed mental picture of what your body will look like when you're at your fittest.

As a helpful hack, instead of asking *what* you want your body to look like, you can simply choose *who* you want to look like. There are a ton of super-fit athletes, celebrities and fitness models out there.

Pick a few guys who already have the body you want and commit yourself to developing it. These are your body avatars and will represent the goal you're working towards.

To get started, go to Google Images or Pinterest and search for the name of your chosen body avatars. You may even want to search for "[body avatar] body" or "[body avatar] shirtless" to find the images that best show off their physique.

WEIRDNESS WARNING!

You may feel weird about this step. (I definitely did.) That's totally natural. In fact, when Googling something like "Hugh Jackman shirtless," weird is probably the right way to feel. Push through the weirdness and do it anyway – I'll explain why in a moment.

Once you've found the images that most inspire you, save them some place where you can refer back to them: either on your computer, in the cloud, or on an image board like Pinterest. It should be a place where you can easily go to see multiple images of the body you're aspiring to build.

Yes, I know it sounds silly. And yes, I know you probably think of vision boards and Pinterest as the tools used by thirteen-year-old girls and moms with hobby blogs. But trust me on this: it works.

I spent three years editing fitness magazines and I can assure you:

frequently looking at pictures of people who have your ideal body type will make you want to get your ass in gear.

Step 2: Find a Workout Plan Geared toward Your Body Avatar

If your body avatars are major celebrities, superheroes or professional athletes, chances are you can simply Google "[body avatar] workout" and find a plethora of results.

You'll obviously want to find a workout that suits your unique needs and will lead to the body type you want. I'm not an exercise physiologist, but a few things to look for in any good workout include:

Variation:

You don't want to do the same thing every time, or work the same muscle groups two days in a row. Look for workouts that mix it up and feature different muscle groups each day. This will help keep you both continually challenged and continually interested.

Enough Leg Exercises:

Too many workouts – especially those based on celebrity bodies – are guilty of focusing on the so-called "glamour" muscles. Don't fall into this trap. You build a body like you build a house: from the ground up. Look for a workout that recognizes the importance of working your legs.

Rest:

Don't worry too much about this one for now, as you're going to adapt any workout you find to suit your schedule. But roughly speaking, workouts that follow a two-days-on / one-day-off pattern work well, especially for beginners.

To get you started, here are a few good workout plans I've found based on commonly Googled celebrities and superheroes. If you're reading this on an e-reader, simply click the links below. If you're going old school and reading the print edition, simply punch the below phrases into Google.

- Hugh Jackman Workout, via Men's Fitness
- Superman Workout, via Muscle and Fitness
- Ryan Gosling Workout, via Fitmole
- Ryan Reynolds Workout via Superhero Jacked
- Captain America Workout, via Bodybuilding.com (This one also offers a nutrition plan.)
- Daniel Craig Workout, via Kinobody.com (Warning: this one's pretty good, but only features one leg day per week.)

Step 3: Plot Out Your Progress

On Sunday, get out a calendar and look at your upcoming week. Planning ahead removes the guessing ("Should I go to the gym today...?") and allows you to adapt your workout plan to your schedule.

Figure out where you can squeeze in workouts throughout the week. I find it helpful to use a weekly planner that breaks down each day hour by hour, as recommended in the classic self-help business book *The 7 Habits of Highly Effective People*. That way, you can plan not just which day you'll workout, but which hour.

Some workout plans will list workouts for Day 1, Day 2, etc., while others will list specific days of the week (chest on Monday, legs on Tuesday, etc.). Don't get too hung up on this.

Don't be afraid to bend your workout plan to your will. It might not be realistic for you to go from working out zero days a week to working out five days a week.

Plan a schedule that you feel good about and think you can realistically stick to. If you feel like you could have done more one week, then tack another workout on to your schedule the following week.

Step 4: Find a Nutrition Plan

Whether you want to build muscle, burn fat or both, nutrition is 80 percent of the equation, especially in the beginning. I'll go into much more detail about nutrition in the next chapter.

Just as you found a workout plan to suit your goals, you need to find an accompanying nutrition plan. Fortunately there are a ton of options out there. I recommend Bodybuilding.com as a pretty good and accessible starting point.

No matter where you find your nutrition plan, there are a few key principles you want to keep in mind; we'll discuss them in detail in the next chapter.

Step 5: Track Your Progress

One of the most effective ways to stick with a training and nutrition regimen is also one of the simplest: write it down.

Take a small notebook with you to the gym and record your results as you go. Depending on your workout, you might record:

- The amount of weight you lift for each set of each exercise
- The amount of time or distance covered on the bike, treadmill or elliptical
- The number of calories you burned
- The amount of rest time you take between each set

Similarly, keep a nutrition journal and jot down what you ate each day. It can be as simple and quick as writing:

- Breakfast: two eggs, toast, coffee
- Morning snack: yogurt with granola and berries
- Lunch: BLT sandwich, donut
- Afternoon snack: apple, walnuts
- Dinner: steak, mushrooms, caesar salad

Step 6: Review Your Progress

Each Sunday or Monday (whichever day you consider to be the start of the week) go back and look at what you achieved during the previous week.

Ask yourself: How can you do just 5 percent better this week? Maybe it's by lifting just two and a half pounds more than last week. Or maybe it's substituting a piece of fruit for a donut just once this week. Focus on small, incremental and easily achievable things you can do to surpass last week's progress.

Over time, these small steps will add up to big results.

TIP:
Focus on what you plan to do (e.g., "I plan to work out three times this week and eat at least six clean, healthy meals"), not on what you want to achieve (e.g., "I want to lose five pounds this week"). Achievements follow actions – focus on the action and the results will follow.

Step 7 (Optional): Be Held Accountable

If you're self-motivated, then all you need to do is keep your journals, reference them, and just "do you." You might not feel comfortable advertising your plans and goals to others (I'm certainly not), and that's totally fine.

But if you're comfortable telling other people what you're up to, it can be extremely motivating to feel like you're accountable to someone else. Whether it's your parents or a close friend, find someone you trust, explain your goals to them and tell them what your plans are for a given week.

Wrapping Up Your Workout Plan

Starting a workout plan doesn't require Herculean effort, just some deliberate action. Use the process laid out in this chapter to get yourself moving and take the first steps toward building a better you.

Of course, if you're going to get yourself in gear you're going to need the right fuel for the job. So in chapter 8, let's explore some ways you can use nutrition to power your progress.

8

EASY WAYS TO EAT CLEAN AND FUEL YOUR GROWTH

"Nutrition is so important. It can't be stressed enough."

– Dwayne Johnson

Starting a workout plan and becoming more active will immediately help you start to feel healthier, happier and more confident in your physical presence. (Eventually you'll also start to look better, though that admittedly comes a little later.) And after reading the previous chapter, I hope you're convinced that it's easier than you might have thought.

But the truth is that if you want to build a strong, healthy body, the gym is not the room you should focus on. As any bodybuilder, professional athlete or movie star bulking up for a role will tell you, bodies are built in the kitchen. So if you want to build more confidence in your physical presence, that's where you've got to start.

Cleaning up your diet will fuel your self-improvement progress by increasing your energy while boosting your immunity –and potentially even your lifespan.

And while nutrition science can be a daunting topic, the basic principles behind it are straightforward and easy to understand. This chapter lays out some guidelines that will help you fuel your training, build the body you want, and increase your overall health.

Eat Fruit for Breakfast

You probably already know that breakfast is the most important meal of the day – and you probably still scarf down a donut, a bagel or some other unhealthy crap, if you eat anything at all.

Starting your day with fruit helps energize you without the accompanying crash that comes from processed sugar or caffeine, and provides an instant hit of vitamins, fiber and healthy carbs, all in one delicious little package.

Plus, research suggests that eating a healthy breakfast will make you more active the rest of the day, which produces all sorts of other downstream benefits, including increased odds that you'll continue eating healthy and get a better night's sleep, to name just two.

Prep Your Meals on Weekends

One of the most effective and confidence-boosting things I've ever done was get into the habit of grocery shopping on Sunday morning and spending the afternoon prepping my meals for the week.

Prepping in advance takes the decision-making – and thus, the unhealthy temptations – out of your meals for the rest of the week. You'll be much more likely to avoid the call of the fast food joint if you've already invested both your time and money into preparing a healthy meal.

Here are a few easy steps to take on Sunday to set yourself up for a healthy week:

1. Buy a pack of boneless, skinless chicken breasts and bake (or better yet, grill) the whole pack, then save the cooked breasts in a Tupperware container in the fridge. You can quickly reheat the chicken and add it to salads or other

dishes all week to ensure you've always got a lean, healthy source of protein on hand.
2. Grab a head of romaine lettuce and chop it up, throw it in a resealable container or bag, then keep it in the fridge too. You can combine it with the chicken for an easy and super healthy salad, or have it as a side with other meals.
3. Buy a bunch of berries (I favor strawberries, blueberries, raspberries and blackberries). Chop up the strawberries, throw them in a strainer with all the others and rinse them well. Put all your mixed berries in a Tupperware and keep it in the fridge. You can add them to oatmeal or shakes throughout the week to add an easy (and delicious) shot of vitamins and nutrients to your snacks.

Live by the Label

Most products nowadays come equipped with a nutritional guide telling you exactly how much sugar, salt, saturated fat and other suspect substances are included in the product.

Get into the habit of checking these labels religiously. Food manufacturers sneak sugar and salt, along with other dubious substances, into everything from bread and pasta sauce to breakfast cereals. You often won't know how much of it you're consuming unless you start checking for yourself and adding it up.

Read the labels of your favorite products, and whenever possible, opt for ones that have less sugar, sodium, saturated fats and other artificial ingredients.

Tip:

As a general rule, if a food is packed full of substances whose names you don't recognize, you probably want to avoid it.

Pack in the Protein

The key to building lean muscle, protein is a must-have nutrient for every man.

A study from the National Institutes of Health has shown that when you consume protein before and after exercise, it not only increases your muscle's ability to recover, but might also help relieve post-workout muscle aches.[18]

And protein's benefits extend even further. Protein fills you up faster than empty carbs, making you less hungry and therefore less likely to give into temptation and fill up on crappy foods.

Protein has also been shown to stabilize blood sugar, ease anxiety and improve cholesterol, among other benefits.[19]

Avoid Protein Bars

While protein is absolutely essential, not all sources are created equal. In fact, some sources are created exceptionally poorly – and then marketed as if they're super foods.

In general, don't waste your money on the protein bars they sell in GNC and other nutrition stores. Yes, they're rich in protein, but they're also packed full of artificial ingredients, including sugar. Some protein bars have as much, if not more, sugar than actual candy bars.

Tip:

Don't be taken in by protein bars that claim to be "sugar-free." These bars often contain sugar alcohols like erythritol and glycerol. Though they do help reduce a bar's calorie count when compared with regular sugar, the trade-off is often more saturated or trans fat.

Instead of snacks full of sugar or fat, opt for natural sources of protein like meat, fish and nuts, and supplement your diet with a sugar-free protein powder that you can mix with fruit, nut milk and other healthy options.

Skip the Sugar

And speaking of the white stuff, you want to avoid it as much as possible.

A growing body of research and evidence suggests that sugar is a particularly toxic chemical responsible for all manner of health deficiencies, including liver disease, metabolic syndrome, type-2 diabetes and even cancer.[20]

Unfortunately, sugar is like the ninja of the junk food world – it sneaks into way more foods than you might expect. Because it's so commonplace in the modern Western diet, it can be difficult to avoid entirely.

But you can still do your health a huge favor by employing some basic common sense. Pass on the foods you know to be rich in the white stuff, like pastries, candy, soda, and fruit juice.

If you really need to get your fix, try replacing candy or other sugar-rich bad habits with a natural source of sugar – namely, fruit. Fruit has enough sugar to satisfy your craving, but it's also got fiber, vitamins and enzymes that help your body process it.

All that healthy stuff is stripped out of processed sugar, which is one of the reasons it's so damn dangerous.

Shake It Up

Making shakes (I refuse to call them "smoothies") is a quick and effective way to combine fruit, vegetables and protein powder into a pretty delicious snack.

If your chief complaint about eating breakfast is that you don't have time in the morning, well, your complaining days may be over, my friend. Whipping up a protein shake is a perfect solution, especially if you make it the night before and keep it in the fridge.

If you don't already have one, pick up a personal-sized blender like a Magic Bullet or a Nutribullet, both of which allow you to easily make shakes that you can take on the go. Now all you need are a couple of recipes so you can make shakes that are nutritious and delicious. Google "protein shake recipes" to find approximately a gajillion – yes, you read that right: a straight-up gajillion!

Avoid the Aisles

You may not have noticed this before, but at most supermarkets, 90 percent of the healthy stuff isn't sitting on a shelf in one of the umpteen aisles. It's usually in some kind of refrigerated area located along the perimeter of the store.

Do a lap around the perimeter of your store and you'll likely pass the produce section, where you should stop and stock up on vitamins and minerals, the butcher and the fishmonger, where you can pick up some lean protein, the dairy section, where you can grab Greek yogurt to add to your breakfast or shakes, and bins full of almonds, cashews and other healthy nuts.

When you hit the grocery store, make this lap before venturing down any aisles. You should only have to pop into the aisles for a few things that will enhance your meals, like condiments and coffee, not for the meal itself.

One word of warning though: even though it's along the perimeter, don't linger too long in the frozen foods section. Those premade meals are stuffed with sodium and other preservatives that neutralize (at best) any health benefits you'd get from the protein or vitamins they might contain.

If you feel like you have to buy frozen for either convenience or cost purposes, remember the Live by the Label guideline and select the ones that have the least sodium.

Drink More Water

The effectiveness of this tactic might be masked by its simplicity, but make no mistake: hydration is immensely important to health.

According to a study by the Centers for Disease Control and Prevention, 78 percent of Americans report drinking less than the recommended eight glasses per day.[21]

That's a problem, because water is imperative for your health. In addition to helping keep you, you know, alive, it also helps fight fatigue, improves your mood, and can stave off headaches, among a whole host of other benefits.

As awesome as water is, don't be taken in by major corporations' (or Jennifer Aniston's) attempts to make you pay for it. The United Nations recognized the right to water and sanitation as a human right back in 2010, and in most corners of the developed world, governments do a pretty good job of making sure that safe, sanitized water flows from your taps.

If you want to go one step further and make sure your water is as pure as possible, invest a small amount in a Brita water filter rather than spend exorbitant amounts of money on bottled water, which carries its own health risks associated with the chemical compound Bisphenol A (BPA) in the bottles, to say nothing of the environmental impact of all that excess packaging.

Assign a Cheat Day

Nobody's perfect, and trying to be will simply set you up for failure. Instead of trying to eat clean seven days a week, pulling it off for a week or two, and then backsliding into the unhealthy abyss, why not set yourself up for long-term success?

Assign one cheat day per week where you're allowed to pig out on whatever you want. Pizza. Cake. Whatever those things Deadpool likes so much are called. (Just kidding. As if pretending to forget the word "chimichangas" would be enough to hide my deep, deep nerdiness.)

Allowing yourself one cheat day per week gives you something to look forward to and something to earn, which will keep you motivated to eat clean for the rest of the week.

And don't fret about whether or not you're setting yourself back by indulging for a day. Eating healthy six days per week and then pigging out one day means that you've got a 6:1 ratio of healthy to unhealthy, which puts you way ahead of the curve.

Final Thoughts on Eating Clean

As Tom Rath, the #1 *New York Times*–bestselling author of *Eat Move Sleep* so succinctly put it: "Eating well does not need to be difficult or complicated. It is possible for healthy eating to be sustainable and even enjoyable."[22]

Follow the guidelines in this chapter to improve your overall nutritional consumption. The increases in energy, health and overall happiness you'll reap as a result will both fuel your progress and provide a significant source of pride that further strengthens your self-confidence.

9

WANT TO STEP UP? REST UP.

"Sleep is that golden chain that ties health and our bodies together."

– Thomas Dekker

I f you really want to become the most confident possible version of yourself, you should really go lie down.

I know, I know. It doesn't sound like the most proactive advice, does it?

And, admittedly, I am exaggerating a little.

What I meant to say is that you should finish reading this chapter, then go lie down. (No one would blame you – my writing tends to have that effect on people.)

Actually, that's not exactly right either. Dropping what you're doing to go take a nap probably won't lead to increased self-confidence. But getting more – and better – sleep definitely will.

The Supremacy of Sleep

A good night's rest is imperative for achieving literally every goal you may want to accomplish while you're awake – including building self-confidence.

"When you lose an hour of sleep, it decreases your well-being, productivity, health and ability to think," writes author and researcher Tom Rath in the aforementioned *Eat Move Sleep*. "Yet people continue to sacrifice sleep before all else."[23]

It's no exaggeration to say that sleep underlies everything that you do. It gives you the energy – and with it, the increased willpower – to eat clean, work out and practice all the other healthy habits that lead to success and personal fulfillment.

But because of its seemingly passive nature, sleep tends to get overlooked as a strategy for building self-confidence. While it might not seem sexy, proactive or all that inspiring, the truth is that regularly getting a good night's sleep is one of the best, most fundamental things you can do to improve your health, happiness and ability to achieve your goals.

Add up all of its benefits, and sleep suddenly becomes a secret weapon for anyone looking to bolster their self-confidence – or any other aspect of their life.

Quality AND Quantity

In order to improve your sleep – and thus, your life – you'll need to focus on both the quality and quantity that you're getting.

An extremely restful slumber isn't going to do you much good if it only lasts an hour. Likewise, blocking out ten hours per night on your schedule will be wasted if you spend much of them tossing, turning and frequently waking up.

The rest of this chapter is dedicated to helping you get both a better and longer night's sleep in order to energize your confidence-building efforts.

Quality: How to Sleep Better

Go Dark

You have evolution to thank for the fact that light is your enemy, at least when it comes to getting a good night's sleep.

For our earliest ancestors, life was pretty simple. It was a whole lot easier to hunt and gather when the sun was out, which made daytime the natural choice for being awake and active. By the time night rolled around, not only were they tired from the day's work, but the light had almost completely disappeared, making it the perfect time to get some rest.

As a result, your body has been programmed to understand that if there's light, you should be awake, and if it's dark, it's time to go to sleep. The trouble, of course, is that unlike our ancestors, today when the sun goes down we're bombarded with myriad sources of artificial light that trick our bodies into thinking we should stay awake.

Whether it's the lightbulbs in our home, the irresistible glow of our TVs, tablets or smartphones, or even the streetlights shining through our windows once we've turned off our own devices, today artificial light is so ubiquitous that it can be hard to signal to your body that it's time to wind down.

Fortunately, there are a few strategies you can use to keep yourself in the dark.

Blackout Blinds

If you live in a city, you probably have light leaking into your bedroom at night from outside, whether from streetlights, billboards, or neighboring buildings that leave their lights on all night.

To combat the bombardment of external light, try using blackout blinds or curtains designed to keep your room pitch black. The darker your room, the easier it will be for your body to know it's time to power down.

Eye Mask

If buying or installing blackout blinds seems like too much of a hassle, try using an eye mask at home while you sleep. Yes, really.

At first, I'll admit, it might feel a little silly. Before I started using an eye mask, I thought of them as nothing more than accessories worn by affected rich people to complement their silk pajamas.

But after using one for a night or two, I was hooked. You don't really notice just how much light is seeping in through your eyelids until you've blocked it out completely. Since making an eye mask a regular staple of my nightly routine, my sleep has been deeper, more restful and more rejuvenating.

Drown Out the Sound

Light isn't the only thing we've evolved to associate with awakeness. Not only did our ancestors slumber peacefully in pitch-black darkness (save for a few stars, of course), they were also unperturbed by the near-constant background noise that plagues our modern ears.

Anyone who lives in a large city knows the familiar hum of cars driving by and honking, construction taking place at seemingly all hours of the night, pedestrians prone to laughing, talking (and sometimes screaming) at all hours, and neighbors whose expensive surround sound systems seem to be set on a timer, programmed to spring to life just as you're winding down.

For us, all this background noise is an inconvenience. But for our ancestors, noise signaled the approach of predators and other potentially life-threatening dangers. As a result, our bodies have evolved to interpret sounds as signals that we should remain awake and alert (lest a saber-toothed tiger snatch you up in the middle of the night).

Plug It Up

If you're more concerned about getting a good night's rest than becoming prey for extinct predators, try using small earplugs. The cheap foam variety sold at pharmacies will work well for most people, or you could look on Amazon for more sophisticated models.

Either way, earplugs help drown out noise and protect your subconscious mind from signals that it might misinterpret as danger, allowing you to rest comfortably knowing that while your neighbor with the surround sound system may be obnoxious, she's no predator.

Quantity: How to Sleep More

While improving your sleeping conditions is important, even sleeping in a pitch-black, soundproof chamber won't do you much good if you're only getting an hour or two of rest each night.

Now that you've learned a few techniques for improving the quality of your sleep, let's go over a few ways you can get more of it.

Fall Asleep Faster

As it turns out, too much light can affect not just the quality of your sleep, as we've discussed, but the quantity too.

Studies have shown that two hours of exposure to light from self-luminous devices like your phone, tablet, computer or TV screen can suppress melatonin, the hormone that regulates sleep in your brain.

That's a problem, since millions of people (myself included) rely on electronic devices for information and entertainment in the evening. Whether it's watching TV on the couch after dinner or taking your tablet or phone to read in bed, your screen has probably become an entrenched part of your evening – and it's a big part of the reason why you toss, turn and can't seem to fall asleep after your head hits the pillow.

How to Stop Staring at the Screen

To ween yourself off your screen and get to sleep faster, try replacing it with a ritual that feels similar, but replaces the ill effects of self-luminous screens with benefits. E-readers like Amazon's Kindle, which you might be using to read this right now, feel similar to other electronic devices but aren't backlit, and therefore don't have the same melatonin-suppressing effect.

Of course you could always go really old school and turn off the TV in favor of perhaps the most surefire method of getting to sleep ever devised by man: reading an actual, honest-to-goodness book. (Remember those?)

Earlier I explained why reading is integral to building self-confidence, but whether you choose an e-reader or a physical book, it's worth noting that a 2009 study from the University of Sussex found reading to be the most effective method for stress reduction.

"Being taken into a literary world eases the tensions in muscles and the heart," as UK newspaper *The Telegraph* reported.

This release of tension puts your body and mind into a calmer, more relaxed state perfect for slumber.

Read More, Rest More

To develop a nightly reading habit, try turning off all your screens half an hour before you would normally go to bed, and start reading instead. Set a goal of reading for half an hour each night for a week. After the first week, turn your screens off half an hour earlier than you did the week before, and read for a full hour before hitting the sack.

Keep upping the ante by a half-hour each week. After a month, you'll have spent a full two hours reading before going to bed, giving your body the time it needs to wind down, and your mind the pleasure of being immersed in a good book.

Stay Asleep Longer

Avoiding screens in the evening will help you fall asleep faster, but wouldn't it be nice if you could extend your sleep a little further in the morning?

Studies suggest that more than 50 percent of people hit the snooze button each day in a desperate (and ultimately ill-fated) attempt to do just that. While this might seem like a great way to extend your sleep, all it really does is throw off your body's natural rhythms and increase the likelihood that you'll feel sluggish all day.

Why is snoozing so detrimental? It has to do with REM. No, not the aging nineties rock band, the other REM – rapid eye movement. REM sleep is the kind that restores and replenishes you, getting you ready for the day ahead. If you go to bed at a decent hour and get enough sleep, you'll usually be coming out of an REM cycle at about the same time as your alarm clock goes off in the morning.

But when you hit snooze and go back to sleep, you re-enter REM – only to be jolted out of it again a scant nine minutes later. Hit the snooze button yet again and you compound your error, making it even harder to shake off the cobwebs when you finally have to get up.

I'm almost embarrassed to confess how guilty of this I used to be. I would calculate the time I absolutely had to get out of bed, then set my alarm clock a full forty minutes earlier than that, just so I could hit snooze a few times before getting up. I basically robbed myself of nearly an hour of restful sleep in favor of frequent, rest-disrupting jolts.

Move the Alarm Clock

You've probably heard the most frequently suggested trick for skipping the snooze button: moving your alarm clock across the room, which forces you to get up. This tactic might sound logical, but in my case, it vastly underestimated just how much I wanted to snooze.

I don't know about you, but my bedroom isn't exactly a cavernous expanse. When I moved my alarm clock from my bedside table to my dresser, I did indeed have to get up and get out of bed to turn it off. But then I looked back at my bed – my warm, plush, inviting bed, sitting just three or four feet away from me – and promptly got back in.

In order to make the "move the alarm clock" trick work, I had to take it one step further: I didn't just move it across the room, but across my condo. I put my alarm clock (by which I of course mean my phone, because obviously) in the bathroom, which is close enough to my bedroom that I can easily hear it, but far enough away that I can't actually see my bed anymore. As soon as I turn off the alarm, I brush my teeth, which further jars me out of my daze and helps me wake up.

It only took a few days for this strategy to stick, and I'm proud to say that I haven't hit snooze in more than a year. And because I actually get up and start my day when my alarm goes off, I no longer need to set it forty minutes early – I remain in a state of restful sleep until I want to get up, and then I do.

Try it for yourself. Move your alarm clock to another room, and then immediately do something that will help keep you out of bed. I like to brush my teeth right away, but you could also chug a glass of water, or, if you have one of those coffee machines with a timer, set it to have a fresh, hot cup waiting for you at the moment you get out of bed.

PART IV

SOLIDIFY YOUR SOCIAL SKILLS

There's simply no denying it: human beings are social creatures.

When you improve your ability to interact with others, you become more confident and at ease in the world – and more fulfilled in the process.

In this part you'll learn a few techniques for overcoming shyness and becoming more comfortable connecting with others. You'll start by learning how to develop, practice and hone your social skills

With that foundation established, next I'll share some hard-won lessons about socializing that took me years to learn for myself, and then reveal a quick trick you can use to dramatically expand your social circles by turning relative strangers into fast friends.

10

COMING OUT OF YOUR SHELL

"You never change your life until you step out of your comfort zone; change begins at the end of your comfort zone."

– Roy T. Bennett

For guys who lean a little more toward the shyer – or even just the more introverted and introspective – end of the spectrum, becoming more comfortable, confident and present around other people is kind of like the Holy Grail.

Interacting with other people may seem intimidating, until you realize that social skills are just like any other skills in that they can be learned, practiced and honed. In this chapter, you'll find out how to start doing all three.

The chapter is divided into three phases: Education, Practice and Honing. The Education phase recommends steps and resources you can use to learn more about socializing norms and techniques. In the second phase, Practice, you'll discover ways you can ease yourself into interacting with people by starting in easy, low-pressure environments. And in the third phase, Honing, you'll start to refine your social aptitude by using your newfound people skills in situations that likely would have intimidated you before.

I speak from experience when I say that for guys who have trouble coming out of their shells, completing this process and becoming more social isn't necessarily easy.

But I also know firsthand that if you commit to it, it can be richly rewarding – and even fun. Once you learn enough to get past your fear and insecurities, you'll quickly realize how enjoyable and enriching it can be to forge connections with your fellow human beings.

So keep an open mind, and enjoy the process.

Phase 1: Educate Yourself

For me, the first step in becoming more social was learning what socializing entailed. How do you start a conversation? How do you keep it going? How do you avoid those awkward moments of silence? Before I could go out to start socializing, my analytical (read: mildly neurotic) mind needed answers to these and many other questions.

I quickly found that unlike other topics, for which good sources of information are scarce, socializing has the opposite problem: there are thousands of books, blogs, podcasts and other resources purporting to tell you exactly how to become socially superior.

The problem, of course, is that not all of them deliver on their promises. I spent far more time and money than I care to admit finding that out the hard way. Only after sifting through a lot of rough did I manage to find a few gems.

To shorten your learning curve, I recommend starting with the six books below – they are easily the best guides I've come across for increasing your social intelligence and confidence.

Tip:

For most of these books, I actually downloaded the audiobook, which I listened to during my commute to work. If you're still struggling to develop the reading habit we discussed in Chapter 6, audiobooks are a great way to learn on the go.

How to Win Friends and Influence People by Dale Carnegie

Written eighty years ago, Carnegie's book holds up so well that today it's regarded as the seminal work on how to interact with humans. Multiple new editions have been released by Carnegie's estate since it was first published, but the book's bread and butter is the fact that his original advice, though anecdotal, stands the test of time.

Carnegie breaks the book into sections that sound like manna from heaven to guys who want to learn how to become more social, such as "Six Ways to Make People Like You," and "Fundamental Techniques for Handling People." Though his claims are lofty, for the most part his advice is sound. This one's an absolute must-read.

How to Talk to Anyone by Leil Lowndes

Author Leil Lowndes may not use the hippest language or make references from this decade (or, to be honest, this century), but this is one of the few books whose subtitle, "92 Little Tricks for Big Success in Relationships," actually delivers. When I was considering reading it, I checked out the Amazon reviews, and was intrigued when I read one that simply said, "This book can make you into a special person." After reading it, I totally agree.

This book has probably done more to improve my social confidence and success than any other resource.

Goodbye to Shy by Leil Lowndes

After reading *How to Talk to Anyone* I was hungry for more from Lowndes, and found this little gem in her catalogue. When learning how to become more social, some guys don't feel like they can dive right into talking to people – they need advice about getting over their own internal hesitation first.

This book does for those guys what the one above does for guys looking to improve their people skills. If you feel too shy, reserved or hesitant to just dive right in and start making small talk, then start here instead.

How to Work a Room by Susan RoAne

Once you've got a few socializing tips under your belt and you're more comfortable talking to people, you can move from merely being comfortable in a room to really working it.

This book is full of good tips that can help you stand out from the crowd. It leans a little professional, providing lots of tips for talking to people at networking events, but it also covers weddings, parties and plenty of other social scenarios in which you're likely to find yourself.

How to Instantly Connect with Anyone by Leil Lowndes

At this point I know what you're thinking, but I swear: I am neither Leil Lowndes' scandalously young lover nor the heir to her estate. I just think her books are really helpful!

Possible May-December romances aside, this one is similar in structure to *How to Talk to Anyone*, but its techniques are a little more ninja. Where *How to Talk to Anyone* is a great way to get conversations (and relationships) started, this one helps you take them to the next level.

The Charisma Myth by Olivia Fox Cabane

If you don't even feel like an adequate socializer, becoming a charismatic one may feel like a bridge too far right now, and I get that. But that's why it's important that you check out Fox Cabane's book. Of its many revelations, the most important may well be this: charisma is something you – yes, you – can turn on and off.

Before I read this, I assumed that charisma was some magic power possessed only by a fortunate few. But Cabane demonstrates that charisma is actually more like a muscle – and this book will teach you how to flex it.

Phase 2: Practice

The great philosopher Kanye West once said, "You gotta crawl before you ball." Likewise, you'll also want to start small and take it slow when developing your people skills.

Many of the books I recommended above offer practice exercises you can use to help you start socializing, which I recommend you try. But if you prefer to ease yourself into things, below are a couple small, easy-to-take steps that will help you feel more comfortable.

None of these is mind-blowingly insightful or complex and that's exactly the point. If you're really struggling to connect with other people, the best way to get over that hump is to start small.

Smile More

Simply smiling at people is one of the most social things you can do, and something of a lost art. Make a point to smile at ten people today while you're walking down the street, out shopping, at the gym, or otherwise just going about your business. It's easy to do, and the reaction you'll get from people will inspire you to do it more.

Give Greetings

After you've smiled at someone, try tossing in a quick "good morning" or "good afternoon." Pleasantries like this could hardly be easier to give, and immediately make people feel acknowledged – which makes it all the more perplexing that few people use them much anymore.

Let society's loss be your gain as you start to sow your sociable oats. (Speaking of things no one says anymore...)

Make Small Talk

I know, I know: small talk sucks. But the truth is that it's easier than you think, and having a series of small, quick and pleasant conversations can go a long way to increasing your social confidence.

To get started, just try commenting on anything around you. If you're in a long line at Starbucks, say "I guess everyone had the same idea" to the person behind you. If you're at the grocery store, ask the cashier how their shift is going and when they get off work. If you're at the mall, wander into a clothing store and ask the store clerk what new styles they have that might work for you.

I'll provide more tips about how to start and sustain conversations in the next chapter, but these tips should be enough for you to find that making small talk is easier than you expected, and people are generally much more receptive to it than you might think – especially if you're already smiling.

Seven Days of Socializing

Try these exercises for a week as you start reading one of the books mentioned in Phase 1.

I'll warn you in advance that if your usual move is to put your headphones on or keep your head down as you plough through people on the way to your destination, then these tactics may feel uncomfortable to you at first.

Push through this discomfort. If you want to achieve a different result, you have to do something different, and trying something new is always going to feel strange at first.

If you do it earnestly, you'll probably find it quickly becomes not just easy, but fun. In fact, I'm willing to bet that you'll keep doing it for more than just seven days.

Phase 3: Honing

At this point you've spent at least a week smiling, chatting and interacting with the people you encounter every day, all while reading some of the best books available about how to improve your social interactions.

It's now time to take things up a notch – don't worry, just one. In this phase you'll start putting some of the socializing techniques you've been learning and practicing to use not with strangers on the street, but with like-minded people with whom you have things in common.

Call Your Friends

Before I started learning how to become more social, I was extremely passive about making plans. I would accept invitations if offered, but rarely would I initiate plans, even with my closest friends.

But calling up some friends for a low-key night out at a restaurant or bar is a great way to put your newly developed social skills into action. The stakes will be relatively low since you're starting with people you're already comfortable with, and you'll find that simply extending an invite and initiating a fun night out provides an immediate boost to your socializing confidence.

This exercise trains you to realize that, nine times out of ten, when you initiate something – be it a conversation, a night out or just about anything else – people are happy to participate.

Plan a Party

A party is the perfect place to hone your socializing skills, and hosting one yourself means that you control the guest list, ensuring that you'll be surrounded by people you know.

Well, mostly.

When you call up your friends for a night out at a bar or restaurant, it usually ends up being just your friends. You'll probably have lots of fun, but you may not even talk to any new or interesting people. Hosting a party, however, makes it much more likely that your friends will bring some friends of their own – which you're going to encourage.

Decide how many people you'd like to have over and invite about 75 percent of that number. Then tell a few of your closest friends that you'd like them to bring friends, so that the rest of the guest list is made up of people you haven't met.

This is a great way to meet and interact with new people, who have essentially been vetted by your friends, in a low-stakes environment in which you're in the driver's seat.

Try a Meetup

If you're ready to move beyond your own social circles, a great place to start is Meetup.com.

Meetup.com is a website where people with similar interests can find each other and arrange to meet in their hometown. They have groups that meet to discuss a whole plethora of topics, from photography to rain dance, from javascript to love for the word plethora. (Alright, fine, I made that last one up.)

Since you'll already have something in common with everyone you meet, conversation will come naturally. This gives you a chance to meet like-minded people and learn how to become more social in an environment you're likely to enjoy.

Join a Sports Team

This one's a no-brainer if your interests tend toward the athletic. Most cities will have a Sport and Social Club that you can join as an individual; the league will then assign you to a team in the sport of your choice.

As with Meetups, you'll already have something in common with the people you'll meet, and more often than not the teams go out for dinner or drinks after the game for some further socializing. It's a great way to exercise both your body and your new social skills.

Go on Some Dates

There's a reason I've left this one for last.

If you're like me, chances are good that you view interacting with potential mates and/or sexual partners as the most intimidating of social situations. But it really doesn't have to be.

Once you've educated yourself, practiced some small talk and further honed your skills in any of the situations listed above, you'll feel much more socially confident. So much so, that you'll even be ready to seek out the people you want to socialize with most.

And thanks to the wonders of the internet, meeting those people is easier than ever. You could of course try a dating app like Tinder, where you and your potential mates will judge each other based almost entirely on your photos. But if you're looking for something a little more substantial, I recommend OkCupid.

OkCupid.com is a free dating site that lets you peruse profiles and send messages to any of its members. This provides you with a low-stakes way of finding potential mates and initiating conversation, because if you send a message to someone and don't get a response, it's no big deal. You can just move on to find someone else who looks interesting. When they do respond, you can trade messages or chat online via instant messenger to establish a rapport, learn more about each other and decide whether you'd like to meet in person.

Trust me when I say I understand how intimidating it is to initiate a conversation – even a digital one – with someone you're attracted to. (In the next chapter I'll explain how I know.)

But after learning more about socializing, arming yourself with a few good conversational tactics and practicing those techniques in a low-stakes environment, talking to people (yes, even attractive people) really can go from intimidating to exciting.

11

WHAT I WISH SOMEONE HAD TOLD ME ABOUT SOCIALIZING

"A man should never be ashamed to own he has been in the wrong, which is but saying... that he is wiser today than he was yesterday."

– Alexander Pope

Anyone who's ever felt nervous before a party knows that socializing can be scary, even after you've gone through the three phases in chapter 10 and started coming out of your shell.

It took me the better part of a decade to figure it out, and while I still I can't claim to be an expert socializer (in fact, I'd be pretty wary of anyone who would make such a claim), I can say with certainty that I have come a long way since my days as a timid and intimidated twenty-one-year-old.

Unfortunately for my younger self, time travel continues to not be a real thing (thanks for nothing, Michael J. Fox), so I can't go back to share my hard-won wisdom with my younger self. But I can help you avoid some of the (many!) mistakes I made, and help make socializing and connecting with others easier, more natural and less intimidating.

In this chapter you'll find twelve lessons about interacting with other people that I wish someone had told me when I was younger, and tips that will help you avoid some common socializing mistakes.

1. Other People Are Shy Too

Part of the reason I found talking to other people so intimidating in my early twenties was I erroneously assumed that I was a below-average socializer.

For some reason, I had this idea in my head that most people were at least average, meaning I saw myself at a constant disadvantage with the majority of people with whom I came into contact.

But the truth was I was so nervous about talking to other people that I retreated into myself. As a result, I largely ignored the thoughts and feelings of others, which prevented me from seeing what a more objective observer would have found obvious: that most of them weren't exactly social butterflies either.

I was so fixated on the (very) small number of people who were actually naturally social, I couldn't see the hundreds of average, introverted and shy people lined up behind them.

Over time I realized that my people skills were actually better than I gave myself credit for; in fact, they were on par with or even above those of many of the people I knew.

This realization immediately made talking to other people less intimidating.

Socializing Tip #1:

You're not the only shy, introverted person – far from it.

Next time you're in a situation in which you have to choose between keeping to yourself or striking up a conversation with a stranger, try to remember that they probably want you to make the first move as much as you want them to.

2. Introversion ≠ Shyness

This is definitely something I didn't know when I was twenty-one. In fact, I didn't actually learn it until I was thirty-one!

It wasn't until I read Susan Cain's book *Quiet: The Power of Introverts in a World That Can't Stop Talking* that I realized just how different introversion and shyness are.

As Cain writes on her website, "Shyness and introversion are not the same thing. Shyness is the fear of negative judgment, and introversion is a preference for quiet, minimally stimulating environments."[24]

What a revelation! For years I felt like some antisocial hermit because I got uncomfortable at big parties or in other stimulating social situations. But I also felt confused, because I loved going to my favorite bars and hanging out with a group of friends, even when that group consisted of a lot of people.

Over the years, my failure to understand how both those things could be true caused me a lot of cognitive dissonance and discomfort.

Learning that it's perfectly possible to be introverted, if not exactly shy, alleviated a lot of anxiety for me. Where was Susan Cain when I was a sophomore?

Socializing Tip #2:

Don't fret too much if you can't understand why some social situations scare you and others don't.

And don't be too hard on yourself if you would genuinely prefer to stay in with a good book rather than go out to some rager.

You're fine, you're normal and you're sure as hell not alone.

3. Extroversion ≠ Superiority

The other great revelation that I got from Cain's book *Quiet* was her notion of the Extrovert Ideal.

In sum, Cain argues that so much of Western culture is built around the notion that being extroverted, outgoing or gregariousness is superior, which naturally leads introverts to think that they are automatically inferior because they lack these qualities.[25]

While Cain doesn't elaborate on the gender-based specifics, in my experience introverted men feel even more burdened by the weight of the Extrovert Ideal and its accordant expectations: men, society would have us believe, are supposed to be the crasser, bolder, more assertive gender.

We frequently watch movies and TV shows where the leading man has no problem talking to women or other strangers, taking charge of a situation and (more often than not) easily charming his way through life.

Naturally we're left with the impression that this is simply how men should be.

But Cain's book is essentially devoted to making the case that this isn't true: introversion is not just "OK" – in many important ways, it's actually awesome.

There are a lot of benefits to being an introvert, including increased self-sufficiency, deeper relationships and a greater appreciation for subtlety and nuance, to name just a few.

Socializing Tip #3:

Don't be taken in by the Extrovert Ideal. Check out Susan Cain's book *Quiet: The Power of Introverts in a World that Can't Stop Talking* to read her compelling argument for introversion in full, and to learn to embrace your introspection.

4. Don't Rehearse Negative Scenarios That Will Never Happen

"I am an old man and have known a great many troubles, most of which never happened."

This quote, often attributed to Mark Twain, gets at an essential truth that many of us can probably relate to: the tendency to imagine negative scenarios that will almost certainly never come to pass.

Negative thinking, of course, can't be eradicated entirely. It doesn't matter if you're the Dalai Lama or Norman Vincent Peale, author of *The Power of Positive Thinking*, everyone succumbs to negative thoughts at one point or another. It's totally natural, and definitely not your fault.

But spending too much time indulging in these negative fantasies is not just useless, it's potentially damaging to your long-term mental and emotional health.

"The more you focus on negativity, the more synapses and neurons your brain will create that support your negative thought process," write Susan Reynolds and Teresa Aubele in *Psychology Today*.[26]

Think of your brain as a sort of sponge: it soaks up what you put into it.

Thinking positively will train your brain to be more positive. Likewise, thinking negatively will prime your brain for negativity, which, as Reynolds and Aubele point out, will slow your ability to process new information, limit your problem-solving capability and negatively impact your mood and impulse control, among other unwanted impacts.

Socializing Tip #4:

Catch yourself in the act. When you realize you're going negative, stop and take a deep breath. Recognize what you're doing, remind yourself that while it's not your fault, it's also not helpful, then redirect your thoughts elsewhere.

Not only will you immediately feel better in that particular moment, but over time you'll find you waste less and less time thinking negatively for no reason.

5. Small Talk Isn't Nearly As Banal As It Seems

I used to get a lot of mileage out of telling myself "I just don't like small talk."

It was too banal, too shallow, too perfunctory. I was better than that, I thought. Deeper. More interested in philosophical discourse than everyday prattle.

As it turns out, I was actually just full of shit.

In my heart of hearts, I knew this was just a lie I told myself to shield my fragile ego from the truth. The real reason I disliked small talk wasn't because it is was banal – it was because I was no damn good at it, and I was infinitely jealous of those who were.

The truth is that small talk isn't petty – it's vital. Think about it. You're not going to have a deep, intellectual conversation with someone who you just met. It takes time to develop that type of relationship; it's something you have to build up to by having a series of smaller, less intimate conversations that allow you to learn more about each other over time.

Small talk is how we both start and build relationships. Sure, it might feel shallow or even disingenuous to talk about the weather, the news or the local sports team. But these low-stakes conversations let you dip your toe into relationship waters and determine whether or not you want to dive in deeper.

Socializing Tip #5:

Don't skip out on small talk because you think it's beneath you. Instead, learn how to get good at it using the techniques mentioned in this book and the ones listed in chapter 10, and marvel at the many new friendships it allows you to form.

6. What You Say Doesn't Matter (Much)

And while we're on the topic of small talk, I've got more good news: it turns out there's really no need to worry about what to say, because the truth is, what you talk about doesn't really matter (much).

This was a tip I first got from the Leil Lowndes book I mentioned earlier, *How to Talk to Anyone*. I read it when I was about twenty-six, but I wish I had learned it a decade or so earlier.

I used to spend so much time fretting about what exactly to say that I ignored an obvious truth: how you say something is just as important – in fact, maybe even more important – than what you say.

Think about the people you most enjoy talking to. Sure, the list may include people who have deep knowledge on a few of your most cherished topics. But I'd be willing to bet that those people only make up a small percentage of your list.

Chances are, the people you most enjoy talking to are the ones who have a friendly cadence and tone, who listen more than they speak and, when they do open their mouths, color almost everything they say with an optimistic, positive, fun or humorous tone.

Becoming aware of this was hugely liberating for me. It relieved me from feeling like I always had to say the "right" thing because it meant almost anything I said would be "right," as long as I said it in an appropriate tone.

Socializing Tip #6:

Worry less about your words. Instead, focus on your tone. Speak in a positive and upbeat cadence, and people will appreciate (almost) anything you have to say.

7. People Love To Talk About Themselves

"Talk to someone about themselves and they'll listen for hours."

This is yet another lesson I learned from Dale Carnegie, the eternal expert in all things human relations and author of *How to Win Friends and Influence People*.[27]

It was as true when Carnegie wrote those words in 1936 as it is today. And much like the wisdom of great philosophers, the beauty of the advice lies in its simplicity.

You can see just how self-evident this essential truth is if you put yourself in the shoes of your conversation partner. Whether you know it (or have admitted it to yourself) before, you probably love talking about yourself whenever you're given the chance: your interests, your hobbies, your accomplishments – just about anything that pertains to you.

And you're not alone. Everyone (myself most certainly included) loves talking about themselves and the things that interest them. Give people a chance to do so and you'll immediately win them over.

Real-World Example:

I was at a party a few years back where a friend of a friend – someone I had never met before – mentioned he had just gotten back from a family vacation to Portugal.

That was all it took to spark a twenty-minute conversation about Portugal, a place I'd never been to and don't have much interest in visiting. (Sorry, Portugal!)

So, how did I keep the conversation going so long? All I did was ask open-ended questions about the trip, a topic I could plainly see he was interested in.

"What was your favorite thing about Portugal? What was the most surprising? What's the weather like at that time of year? How was the food? They make some wine there too, don't they?"

By giving him a chance to talk about his trip and his passion, I not only got to know him better and established a connection, I was able to leave him with a positive impression of me.

And I barely had to open my mouth.

Socializing Tip #7:

Give people a chance to talk about themselves and their interests, and really listen as they answer.

8. Smiles Are Everything

I mentioned a few of the benefits of smiling back in chapter 10, but this little strategy is so shockingly effective that it bears exploring a little further.

In short, smiling makes almost every social situation better.

For instance, smiling can make you seem more approachable. As Alyssa Detweiler writes on Inspyr.com, "Studies have found that people are more willing to engage socially with others who are smiling."[28]

And the benefits don't end with increased approachability.

"A smile suggests that you're personable, easy going, and empathetic," Detweiler continues. "In fact, a study in the *European Journal of Social Psychology* found that smiling actually makes you more attractive to those you smile at."

As if that weren't enough reason to grin, smiling has been shown to provide significant benefits to both your brain and your body.

Smiling helps you manage stress, relax your body and lower both your heart rate and blood pressure, according to Sarah Stevenson in *Psychology Today*.

"Each time you smile at a person, their brain coaxes them to return the favor," says Stevenson.

"You are creating a symbiotic relationship that allows both of you to release feel good chemicals in your brain, activate reward centers, make you both more attractive and increase the chances of you both living longer, healthier lives."[29]

And here you thought smiles were just upside-down frowns.

Socializing Tip #8:

Smile more. At first it may seem weird to make a conscious point of smiling, but do it anyway. You'll instantly feel better about yourself, and make other people feel good too.

9. Inaction Is Way Worse Than Awkwardness

I didn't date much in university. Actually, I should clarify.

It would be more accurate to say I only went on a small number of dates in university.

In fact, that's not quite accurate either.

It would be most accurate to say that I only went on the smallest number of dates possible in university.

Which is to say, the number of dates I went on is... one.

It's not that I didn't have opportunities. Over the years there were plenty of girls I was interested in, and even a scant few who expressed some interest in me. It's just that I was terrified of going on a first date, and everything that would entail.

What the hell would I talk about? What's the proper etiquette? Do I pick her up, or do we meet somewhere? Do I walk her home? Do I kiss her at the end? Will she even want me to kiss her at the end? How will I know?

I was so afraid of awkwardness that I never asked out a single girl. (In case you were wondering about the lone date that I did go on, the girl actually asked me out.)

So to avoid going on awkward dates, I went on no dates. Instead, I sat at home with my roommate, playing video games and pining over the social life I could have had, but didn't.

Real-World Example:

My early dating experiences were... less than stellar, let's say.

Fortunately, after university I moved to a big city. I didn't have a roommate anymore, and thus, no one to hang out with and use as an excuse for not going out to meet new people. So after years of inaction I finally created an online dating profile and started putting myself out there.

And, yep: shit got awkward.

In my earliest dips into the dating pool, I was not a good date. I struggled to come up with date ideas, didn't know what to say and generally just stumbled through the whole thing. On more than one occasion I was so nervous beforehand that I almost cancelled before we met up.

But I didn't cancel. I resolved to keep going on first dates, awkward though they were, until they got easier.

And it worked... eventually.

Over time I got better, more comfortable, even confident on a date. It wasn't easy. And sometimes it wasn't even all that fun. But it was a hell of a lot better than staying home and playing video games on a Saturday night.

Socializing Tip #9:

Don't avoid social situations because you're afraid that they'll be awkward. They will be awkward – at least at first.

But the only way to make them less awkward is to practice them.

Again and again and again.

10. You Can Fake It 'Til You Make It (Sort Of)

I know, I know: this is one of those jargony self-help sayings that sounds suspiciously like bullshit. But you don't need a degree in psychology to know that it's true. You just need to have experienced it for yourself.

My dating experience above is a great example. On those first few dates, I didn't know what the hell I was doing, and it showed. But over time I started to learn a little bit more about how to be a good date. It still totally terrified me, but at least I had some idea what I was doing.

This led me to feel like I could do it, which in turn made me less terrified. And eventually I went from *feeling* like I could do it to *knowing* I could. After that, going on dates actually became fun.

Now, don't get me wrong: I'm definitely not advocating that you pretend to be someone you're not. (In the next tip, you'll find out why.) But I am saying that if you follow the previous tip and take action – even action that puts you outside of your comfort zone – you'll find that it gets easier each time.

And as a result, you will get better and better at socializing – or anything else you're trying to achieve.

Socializing Tip #10:

Fake it 'til you make it. Put yourself out there and resolve to keep doing so until you get better – at small talk, at dating, at going to parties, or whatever it is you want to achieve.

11. It's Easy To See Through Phoniness

Remember earlier when I described the dread I used to feel when I went to parties? What I didn't tell you was how I acted after I finally mustered up the courage to go.

I played it totally cool. I did a super-sweet cool guy lean against whatever flat surface was available, looked brooding and mysterious while not saying much, and left everyone there with the impression that I was deep, soulful, enigmatic and alluring.

And if you believe that, I've got a great real estate opportunity on Mars for you.

In truth I probably looked more like Zach Braff in *Garden State*. Remember that scene where he's literally wearing a shirt made from the same fabric as the wallpaper, so that he seamlessly blends right in?

Yeah, that was basically me. Or at least, that's how I felt. And as much as I would have loved to believe that I was hiding my wallflower feelings behind a finely crafted mask of mystery and bravado, the truth is that everyone could see right through it.

And if you're doing something similar, they can see through you, too.

Instead of pretending I was totally cool, I would have been way better served if I admitted my awkwardness, even if I couldn't quite bring myself to embrace it.

I know it's tough, but ultimately, it's better to be the guy who's shy but earnest than the guy who's shy and desperately trying to hide it.

Socializing Tip #11:

Don't try to mask your shyness or introversion by acting brooding or mysterious. You won't come off as cool, you'll come off as insincere and insecure, which is exactly what you're trying to avoid.

12. Grow Your Social Circle To Grow Yourself

When I first went to university, I was so afraid to meet new people that I told myself yet another comforting lie: "I have enough friends."

Like most good lies, it had a hint of truth to it; I did indeed have a lot of great, close friends, for whom I felt really grateful.

But with the benefit of hindsight, it's become obvious that I was just fixating on this truth as a way to avoid another, far less comforting one: that talking to people and making new friends intimidated the hell out of me.

Thankfully, I had no choice but to ditch the whole "I have enough friends" lie.

Because, while I did have some great friends in high school, not a single one of them went to my university – which meant that my only two options were to make some new friends or prepare myself for an extremely lonely (to say nothing of boring) four years.

And thank God I did. By opening myself up to new people I expanded not only my social circle, but my horizons. I met people from all walks of life and corners of the globe who taught me about themselves, their passions and the worlds they came from.

My life is far richer, happier and more fulfilling because of these people. I hate to think where I'd be if I hadn't forced myself to embrace them.

Socializing Tip #12:

Remain open to meeting new people and making new friends. Yes, it can sometimes be intimidating. But it's also richly rewarding. Don't let your fear keep you from enjoying one of life's great pleasures: developing real, lasting bonds with other people.

When you start applying the tips you've learned in this chapter, you'll quickly come to find that interacting with other people is a lot less intimidating and nerve-racking when you have a few socializing tricks up your sleeve.

And the best part is that consciously employing a few proven tactics will not just make you feel more comfortable – it will make you more friends.

In the next chapter, I'll share one of my favorite strategies for turning new acquaintances into fast friends.

12

A QUICK TRICK FOR MAKING FAST FRIENDS

"Lay this unto your breast: Old friends, like old swords, still are trusted best."

– John Webster

Kyle was one of those guys who got along with everyone.*

A senior director at the company where I used to work, Kyle was one of the few people who seemed to rise above, or at least exist outside of, office politics.

It didn't matter if he annoyed you with lame jokes (which he did), failed to return your emails promptly (if at all) or straight up told you to "f*ck off!" (his greeting of choice) as soon as you entered his office. He somehow managed to make it all endearing, and as a result he could count nearly every person in the office as an ally, and many as close personal friends.

As someone who was raised to be incessantly polite, I've always been envious of guys like Kyle. How is it that a guy who does whatever he wants all the time could, simultaneously, win over so many people?

The question plagued me for months, so I started watching Kyle more closely to see if I could come up with any clues. To be sure, he had much better social skills than his brash personality would have you believe. He might yell "f*ck off!" when you walked in his office, but if you stayed to talk about a work-related issue, he'd follow up by making time to ask about your week, your family, your upcoming vacation, etc.

But this fact alone didn't explain it. You could ask the most flattering questions in the world, but you're not going to win many points with your conversation partner if you precede your questions with a rousing "Go f*ck yourself" as you stare them dead in the eyes. After all, you only get one chance to make a good first impression.

A few confounding months later, the answer finally became clear. Kyle didn't work in my department, but he would frequently come over to "visit," by which he meant chat about the news or what we were watching on TV in order to kill time before he had to go back to his desk.

One week a new employee started in my department, placing her squarely in the middle of Kyle's usual time-killing conversation circle.

The next time Kyle came to chat with my colleagues and me, we all launched into our usual spiel about our favorite TV show as our new hire sat there somewhat awkwardly, clearly feeling like an outsider stuck on the inside of a conversation.

That's when Kyle performed one of the most masterful socializing techniques I've ever witnessed. It would have been so easy to either ignore our new colleague, or unintentionally interrogate her and put her on the spot – "Do you watch the show we all love?" Instead, he said something so ingenious that I still find myself in awe.

So, what was this master stroke of socializing that continues to marvel me? Kyle simply turned to our newest colleague and asked, in his usual calm but somewhat incredulous tone, "Wasn't that last episode total shit?"

In one fell swoop, he skipped right past the preamble, the pleasantries and the awkward "getting to know you" phase that 99 percent of people engage in when they meet someone new. Instead, he immediately started treating our newest colleague like an old friend.

Let me repeat that: he immediately started treating her like an old friend.

Old friends don't ask, "So, do you like [insert topic of conversation here]?" They don't speak in a superficially friendly tone. And they don't bother with sussing out each other's likes and dislikes in order to avoid saying anything offensive.

Old friends dispense with all the pleasantries and cut right to the chase – "Wasn't that last episode total shit?" – and in so doing, they make each other feel known and connected, like they're part of a shared tribe.

For Kyle, there was nothing to lose and everything to gain by phrasing the question that way. If she didn't watch the show, she would just say, "I don't know, I don't watch it." But if she did, she could respond with her own thoughts on the episode, and immediately feel like one of the gang – which is exactly what happened.

As I reflected more on this maneuver, I remembered back to my first interaction with Kyle and realized he had done the same thing with me.

On my first day, he was out of the office, so we didn't meet. The following day, my boss and I bumped into him in the kitchen, and she introduced us. Instead of offering me the same "Hi, welcome aboard" that everyone else had given me, he said, "Oh yeah, I missed you yesterday – I've been meaning to ask how the first day went." Then he continued conspiratorially, "Who made the worst first impression?"

While I wasn't conscious of it at the time, when I looked back on it I realized how much that had endeared me to Kyle. Not only did he stand out from the other new colleagues I had just met, but he immediately made me feel like he and I shared a secret that no one else was in on.

Just like old friends.

Your Move: Treat New People like Old Friends

You can utilize Kyle's strategy to make new people you meet feel like you've been friends for years.

Next time you meet a new colleague, classmate, friend of a friend or anyone else who's already somehow a part of your sphere, dispense with all the pleasantries and start treating them like a member of your tribe from the get-go.

Do them a favor that you would normally only do for someone you know well. Share some of your likes and dislikes without pausing to worry about how you'll be perceived. Or learn from Kyle and just ask them a question as nonchalantly as you would ask an old friend.

Pretty soon, they'll be one.

PART V

STRENGTHEN YOUR STYLE

Clothes don't make the man – but they can sure as hell make him feel confident.

When you look good, you feel good, and the better you feel the more likely you'll be to take action in other important areas of your life.

That's why this final part is devoted to exploring the ways you can use style to strengthen your self-confidence. First, we'll explore the science that connects looking good to feeling good. With that understanding established, you'll next learn how to cultivate a unique, dapper look that you can be proud of, and then discover how to really take your look next level by using a few handsome hacks designed to help any man look (and feel) his best.

13

THE LINK BETWEEN STYLE AND SELF-CONFIDENCE

"Clothes and manners do not make the man; but when he is made, they greatly improve his appearance."

– Arthur Ashe

Have you ever seen that movie with Ryan Gosling and Steve Carell?

No, not the one about Wall Street where Carell wore that ridiculous blonde wig.

I mean the first one: *Crazy, Stupid, Love.*

In it, Steve Carell plays a guy who finds out that his wife has been cheating on him, which leads to an existential crisis as he spirals into self-doubt and despair.

Ryan Gosling, meanwhile, basically plays Ryan Gosling. His character is a swaggering lothario with seemingly unshakeable self-confidence – and, interestingly, a heart of gold – who decides to take Carell's character under his wing and help him bounce back from his depression.

And where's the very first place Gosling's charismatic character takes Carell to regain his mojo?

The (mothafuckin') mall.

In the grand tradition of movie characters like Danny Ocean, James Bond and Thomas Crown before him, Gosling's character understood that one of the best, most immediate and effective ways to feel better on the inside is to look better on the outside.

If you've ever pulled on a suit jacket that fit you like a glove and looked in the mirror as you buttoned it up, you'll know that the clothes you wear (and the rest of your overall look) have an undeniable effect on the way you feel.

Tucking in a crisp white dress shirt makes you feel professional and deft.

Knotting your tie feels courtly and dignified.

And buttoning up a well-fitting jacket makes you stand up taller and carry yourself with pride.

Fortunately for those of us who don't work in the financial industry or star in the hit show *Suits*, you can get the same kind of instant, confidence-boosting feeling even without suiting up.

The same self-esteem-bolstering effects extend to any piece of clothing that makes you feel poised, polished and put together.

The Halo Effect

Since the days of Helen of Troy, whose beauty launched a thousand ships, it's been understood that attractive people have a certain advantage when it comes to, well, just about everything.

"In society, attractive people tend to be more intelligent, better adjusted, and more popular," writes Stanford University's Charles Feng in the *Journal of Young Investigators*.

"Research shows attractive people also have more occupational success and more dating experience than their unattractive counterparts."[30]

Scientists call this "the Halo Effect," because good-looking people just seem so damn perfect that our gut reaction is to compare them to angels.

Now, on the off chance that you weren't born with the genetic makeup of a young Brad Pitt, I can understand how this would sound discouraging.

Just as the rich tend to get richer, the hot tend to get hotter – oh, plus they get all the wealth, friends and dating partners.

FML, right?

Wrong, actually.

Projecting Confidence

As Feng explains, there actually is a way for those of us who look less like Brad Pitt and more like Brad Garrett to get in on the Halo Effect:

"Elliot Aronson, a social psychologist at Stanford University, believes self-fulfilling prophecies – in which a person's confident self-perception, further perpetuated by healthy feedback from others – may play a role in success as well," Feng writes.

"Aronson suggests, based on the self-fulfilling prophecy, that people who feel they are attractive… are just as successful as their counterparts who are judged to be good-looking."[31] Essentially, as long as you truly and authentically *feel* like you look good, you'll project that feeling outward to other people.

In turn, people will then treat you the same way they would treat any other good-looking person. And the best part is that this creates a positive feedback loop, because you then interpret the positive treatment you're receiving as confirmation that you do indeed look good – which in turn makes you feel even better.

So, even if you didn't win the genetic lottery, you can get all the same benefits that good-looking people enjoy by dressing and presenting yourself well.

As reasons to tuck in your shirt go, that's a pretty damn good one.

But, wait a second, let's pause here and acknowledge that this is all a little vain, isn't it?

I mean, sure, it's nice to look good, but it's not exactly essential. Surely there are other more important (to say nothing of more benevolent) pursuits when it comes to building our self-confidence.

Well, yeah.

But not as many as you might think.

A Positive Paradox

One of the most important lessons I've learned in my years of researching, writing about and building self-confidence is that one of the best things you can do to increase your own confidence is to not focus on yourself at all, but on other people.

Doing something kind for another person is, somewhat paradoxically, one of the best ways to feel better about yourself.

But the paradox goes even deeper than that.

As it turns out, one of the best ways to increase the likelihood that you'll do something kind for another person – and thus, feel better about yourself – is to focus on making yourself feel better first.

At this point you'd be completely forgiven for thinking that what started out as a simple chapter about a sweet-ass Ryan Gosling movie has declined into psychological mumbo jumbo.

But I swear it's not quackery, it's science.

This is another concept pioneered by Nathaniel Branden, the psychologist and author of *The Six Pillars of Self-Esteem*, who you met way back in chapter 1.

"There is overwhelming evidence that the higher the level of self-esteem, the more likely one will be to treat others with respect, kindness, and generosity," Branden writes.[32]

So looking good leads to feeling good, and feeling good leads to helping people, and helping people leads to... well, feeling good.

Let's break it down in a little more detail.

How Looking Good Leads to Doing Good

1. Doing nice things for other people makes you feel good
2. According to Branden, you'll be more likely to perform these kind acts if you already feel good about yourself
3. Since looking good is a great and relatively easy way to

make yourself feel good, doing things that make you look better can also make you more likely to help others
4. Once you start helping people, you'll feel even better about yourself, which will in turn make you even more likely to continue doing it

When you look at it like that, dressing and presenting yourself well turns out to be not so much a paradox, but a path – to kindness, generosity, respect and, of course, self-confidence

In this light, it's no wonder that Ryan Gosling's confident and charismatic go-getter took down-in-the-dumps Steve Carell under his wing: helping Carell become more confident also helped Gosling feel more confident in the process.

Your Confidence Compounds

There's good reason to believe that looking good is one path to self-confidence, but it's also important to note that it's not the only one.

As we've already established, building a well-rounded sense of self-confidence means improving not just your style, but your mind, body and people skills (among other things), and not always in equal measure.

When I'm trying to develop a new healthy habit, I devote more time to cultivating the right mindset. If I'm trying to reach a new goal at the gym, I'll focus more on my body. When I know I have a party or social event coming up, I'll spend some time making sure my conversation skills are well honed. And back when I was single and looking for a relationship, I made sure to learn the finer points of dating and attracting a partner.

But one of the best parts about starting to build self-confidence is that you quickly realize that improving in one area pays dividends in many others. So as you take steps to improve your style and your overall look, you'll likely find yourself more motivated to improve your mind, body, people skills and other facets of your life, too.

Like I said: not a bad reason to tuck in your shirt, right?

14

CREATING A PERSONAL STYLE PROFILE

"Being perfectly well-dressed gives one a tranquility that no religion can bestow."

– Ralph Waldo Emerson

What does self-confidence look like?

As with many of life's great questions – Why are we here? What does it all mean? Why do people keep letting Adam Sandler make movies? – the query may sound simple, but the answer is deceptively more complex.

For instance, if you Google "what does a confident guy look like" you'll find that the world's greatest search engine seems to think self-confidence means putting on a suit and adjusting your shirt cuffs in a stock photo.

Now, don't get me wrong – I'm all for suiting up and making sure your shirt cuffs are on point. But I also know that not everyone feels comfortable wearing a suit, or constantly fidgeting with his wrists for no discernible reason.

And there's a reason why even Google's algorithm can't quite nail down what self-confidence looks like: because it looks different to everyone.

Sure, there are some fundamental body language cues that convey power, dominance and confidence to the reptilian side of our puny human brains, and it can be helpful to understand what those are and how they work.

But if you're looking to give your own confidence a boost through what you wear, then you don't need to ask Google what confidence looks like, you need to ask yourself. (And yes, I know that sounded kind of like a fortune cookie – but it's true!)

Your Personal Style Profile

One of the best ways I've found to look more confident is by creating and adhering to what I call a Personal Style Profile.

"Hey Dave, quick question: what the hell is a Personal Style Profile?"

– You, just now

Great question, you.

A Personal Style Profile is essentially a template for your style. It's the underlying, fundamental framework that makes it easy to assemble your wardrobe, choose your haircut or navigate any of life's myriad other style dilemmas.

Your Personal Style Profile is the paradigm in which you feel the most comfortable and confident.

Let me put it this way:

Imagine a good friend of yours is describing you to someone you've never met. The stranger asks your friend, "How does he dress?"

Your friend, of course, isn't going to describe every item of clothing you own. They're going to give a broad, shorthand description that captures the essence of your style and allows the stranger to paint a picture in their head.

What two or three words would you want your friend to use to describe you?

Maybe it's something like "Don Draper–esque." Or you might be going for a "modern cowboy" look. Or maybe it's "fashion-forward scientist," "Japanese DJ," "Savile Row gentleman," "K-Pop all star," "hillbilly hipster," "CEO-chic" or any of a thousand other possibilities.

Your Personal Style Profile, then, is whatever fashion, style or archetype most inspires you; it's the overall look that makes you feel the most comfortable and confident.

Why Define a Personal Style Profile?

The truth is that whether you take the time to define your profile or not, you've got one.

Though some of us may spend more time thinking about how to look confident than others do, we all have certain influences and style inclinations that we associate with confidence.

Exactly whose style you're influenced by will of course be unique to you and your own situation. But no one lives in a bubble and no one is immune to these influences.

Your own Personal Style Profile may stem from authority figures in your life, movie stars you see on screen, your colleagues and peers, or any of umpteen other sources. But one way or another you've developed some sense of what you think confidence looks like.

Taking time to devote deliberate thought to this will help crystallize it in your mind and come up with an overall look that feels authentic and comfortable – both of which go a long way toward answering the question of how to look confident.

This can be a personally revealing exercise too, as it forces you to question your influences and determine which of them you truly want to emulate. What look really speaks to you on a visceral, gut level?

Do it Once, Do it Right

While determining your Personal Style Profile may require a little thought and effort, the good news is that, in all likelihood, you'll only have to do it once.

The Profile is meant as a template, a broad and overarching set of guidelines, rather than a blueprint, which is specific and precise.

Throughout your adult life you'll no doubt go through hundreds of different pieces of clothing, and your tastes will vary over time. You'll also likely go through phases where you prefer one look over others, for better or worse. (Many of my friends still revel in reminding me that my sweater vest phase was decidedly for worse.)

But in all likelihood, you're not going to make too many wholesale changes to your Personal Style Profile – not many guys switch from the "Wall Street titan" look to "modern goth," after all – so chances are good that once you put in the time to define your profile, it can guide you for the rest of your life.

How a Personal Style Profile Can Save You Money

Taking the time to define your Personal Style Profile may seem like an unnecessary chore, but it's actually more like an investment.

In one sense, it's a monetary investment. I don't know about you, but in my younger days I wasted a lot of money on clothes I erroneously thought I had to have.

Sometimes I would see a certain look in a movie and just get obsessed with it. On other occasions, I would let salespeople talk me into shit I knew deep down I didn't need or wouldn't really work for me.

But now that I have a well-defined Personal Style Profile, shopping is a lot easier. Do I still sometimes make impulse purchases? My closet packed full of blue shirts in very slightly different shades would suggest that yes, I still do.

But I no longer buy things that I'm only going to wear once or twice or get tired of after just a few months. In fact, I never buy a piece unless I know how I'm going to wear it and that I can reasonably expect to get at least a few years' worth of use from it.

How a Personal Style Profile Can Save You Time

And my Profile hasn't just saved me untold dollars, it has saved me a ton of time.

Previously I would indecisively wander around a mall or department store for hours. I would stop and try on a few things, hesitate and debate whether or not I should buy it, then repeat this process in two, three or four other stores.

Did I want a super-badass motorcycle jacket or a friendly and approachable cardigan? Would I drop a few hundred dollars on leather dress shoes or just pick up a pair of Chucks and embrace my inner skater?

And then once I made up my mind, I would have to start the deliberations all over again to choose a color!

No more. Now that I know my Personal Style Profile, I can tell right away whether or not a piece is in my wheelhouse. And while I do try to diversify my color options, I also know that there are some colors that just don't fit with the look I'm going for. (Sorry, pink. It's not you, it's me.)

Personal Style Leads to Personal Confidence

Because I now have a dresser and closet full of clothes that were specifically chosen because they fit my own Personal Style Profile, I know that I can look and feel my best every time I leave the house.

Even if I'm wearing a sweater vest.

Creating Your Personal Style Profile

To guide you through the creation of your own Personal Style Profile, I've created a (totally free!) ten-step checklist.

Simply check out my website, www.IrreverentGent.com/Personal-Style-Profile, to download it and start defining your most dapper look.

15

HANDSOME HACKS TO HELP YOU LOOK YOUR BEST

The (handsome) devil is in the details.

At this point we've already covered the big, life-changing investments you can make in order to look and feel better over the long haul.

Starting a workout plan, cleaning up your diet and defining your Personal Style Profile are all fundamental steps to cultivate a look that you can be proud of today and for years to come.

But as a wise and articulate philosopher once so astutely noted, "Ain't nobody got tiiiiiime for that."

Fair enough, you noble scholar you.

If you want to start looking better right away, there are a number of quick and easy ways to work with what you've already got.

Will these tips alone turn you into a *GQ* cover model overnight? Probably not. For that, you'll have to invest your time into the larger, more life-changing efforts mentioned above.

However, when it comes to refining your look, a little goes a long way; you'd be surprised how much you can move the needle just by nailing the details and doing a bunch of little things right.

So take a look at the handsome hacks in this chapter, decide which ones feel right for you, then implement as many as you can. When it comes to refining your look, a little goes a long way.

1. Ditch Your Razor (and Get a Beard Trimmer)

It's a scientifically proven fact: chicks dig facial hair.

In a study published in the *Journal of Evolutionary Biology*, women were shown a man's face in various states of beardedness, from clean-shaven all the way up to full Grizzly Adams. The results? "Stubble was judged as most attractive overall," according to the study.[33]

Interestingly, full beards were judged more attractive for long-term relationships than short-term ones, but in all cases, men with clean-shaven faces ranked the lowest.

Your Move:

Stop shaving your face. Instead, use a beard trimmer that will leave the perfect amount of stubble.

I've been using the Wahl Lithium Ion for a year now and absolutely swear by it. In addition to looking sleek and sexy itself, it leaves a perfect amount of stubble every time, with no razor burn or bumps.

2. Get Rid of Unsightly Body Hair

On second thought, don't throw that razor away just yet.

While stubble or a well-kept beard might help you land a date, no one has ever said, "Wow, look at all his sexy back hair."

Keep yourself well groomed in the areas of your body that are most likely to peek out from underneath your collar or sleeves.

If you live in a warm climate or taking a beach-bound vacation, this rule extends to any body part that will be seen when you pop your shirt off (think shoulders, upper arms, lower back, etc.).

Your Move:

Use a razor and some shaving cream to get rid of unflattering shoulder, back and neck hair.

3. Go Pluck Yourself

This is one of those things that Hollywood stylists swear by, but the average guy doesn't often think about. You may not give your eyebrows much thought, but apparently women do.

"Your eyebrows are one of the first things we notice, besides that amazing smile, of course," writes Huffington Post Fashion and Beauty Editor Dana Oliver.[34]

Our eyebrows? Who knew!

Women, apparently. As guys we tend to focus on the more basic grooming measures like brushing our teeth and combing our hair, but as it turns out, the (handsome) devil is in the details.

Once you become aware of how much eyebrows affect attractiveness, you'll start noticing how really handsome guys – like, say, Hollywood's leading men – almost always have impeccable brow game.

For a case study, look no further than former comic relief and current Guardian of the Galaxy Chris Pratt.

Pratt famously got in superhero shape for his role in *Guardians of the Galaxy*, and there's no denying that the extra muscle he packed on (and the square jaw that was apparently hiding under Andy Dwyer's baby fat) are what helped propel him into leading-man status.

But once he was there, Hollywood stylists apparently let him in on the eyebrow secret. Google any photo of Chris Pratt on the promotional circuit for *Guardians* to see what I mean.

The goofy Chris Pratt, the one we got to know way back on shows like *Everwood* and *Parks and Recreation* didn't exactly have a unibrow, but his eyebrows were clearly untamed and kind of disheveled. Which is to say, exactly like yours and mine.

But the handsome-ass Chris Pratt who seduces Zoe Saldana and Jennifer Lawrence in blockbuster movies? His eyebrows are clearly better groomed and more controlled than those of his younger self, and as on point as his fitness, style and skin tone (more on that later).

Your Move:

Pick up a grooming kit and use the tweezer and tiny scissors to remove any stray hairs along the edges of your brows – and especially, of course, the ones in the middle above the bridge of your nose.

But for the love of god, do *not* overdo it. You're going for Chris Pratt, not Snooki from *Jersey Shore*.

4. Whiten Your Teeth

Speaking of grooming tricks you might not think of, when was the last time you gave much thought to your chompers?

It's easy to forget about them, but everybody else sees your teeth every time you open your mouth. So it's in your best interest to keep them looking clean, well cared for and at least close to a normal shade of white.

Your Move:

Find the teeth-whitening method that's right for you.

Personally I like to use whitening toothpaste in order to combat the daily deluge of teeth-yellowing coffee I subject my mouth to. I've also had good results from the occasional use of Crest White Strips and other at-home whitening kits.

For best results, consult your dentist about which method will work best for you.

5. Rock a New Haircut

It's no secret that men are creatures of habit, and nowhere is this more plainly evident than on the top of our heads.

Most guys have some variation of the same haircut for years and even decades, giving little thought to one of our most noticeable features. But by ignoring your hair, you're missing out on a golden opportunity to elevate your look.

A well-chosen and well-styled look on top can make an otherwise "meh" visage look put together, refined and handsome.

Your Move:

Google "best men's haircuts" and find a few pictures that strike you. Save them on your phone and take them into your barber to give them an idea of what you're going for. They'll help you adapt the look to your head shape.

6. Use Less Hair Product

Your barber can only do so much. Once you've found the haircut that works for you, it's up to you to style it properly.

This is a mistake a lot of young guys make, and I have to admit that I was especially guilty of it back in the day.

As a kid who grew up in the nineties—when both the boy band era and TV's *Friends* were at their pinnacle—I used to think I needed to gob product into my hair by the handful.

Sometimes my hair looked like one of those plastic cheese graters. As a general rule, anytime a part of your body looks like it could carve off pieces of Parmesan, you've got a problem.

By contrast, flip through men's magazines like *GQ* and *Esquire* and take a close look at the hair of their models.

Is there some product in there? Probably – it's hard to maintain that "windswept" look without actual wind. But did they overdo it? Almost never.

Their hair looks both stylish and natural, which is perfect for any style short of a tuxedo.

Your Move:

Don't overdo it on the hair product. Try using just one finger when you scoop it out of the jar, then apply it and style it appropriately.

This method will help keep you from gobbing on too much. You can always dip back in if you decide you need a little extra.

7. Clip Your Nails

Remember that grooming kit you bought after learning about the magic of maintaining your eyebrows?

It came with a nail clipper, and you need to use it.

Whereas you might have a (totally understandable and perfectly legitimate) argument for why plucking your eyebrows is one step further than you're willing to travel on the road to Handsometown, there's absolutely no excuse for neglecting your nail-trimming duties.

No one's saying you have to go get a manicure. Though if you do, no one's going to judge you for it, either. (You do you, my friend.)

But for the love of God, don't let your claws grow out of control.

Your Move:

Use a nail clipper to trim your nails regularly.

8. Try Self-Tanner

(Yes, seriously. Just hear me out.)

For the final grooming tip of the chapter, I've saved what's undoubtedly the weirdest for last.

This one comes courtesy of fashion-world kingpin Michael Kors, who told *GQ* in 2013, "A tan makes you look healthy. My secret is Jergens self-tanning moisturizer. Gives you just a bit of color."[35]

Now before I go any further, let me pause and acknowledge how bat-shit crazy this advice probably sounds. We're dudes! We don't bother fretting about our tans, right?

Well, maybe we should. A study done at the University of Toronto examined the skin tone of male and female models. White male models had skin that was 15 percent darker than white female models, while the skin of black male models was 11 percent darker than their female counterparts.[36]

Why do most male models have darker skin? Because women are apparently predisposed to finding darker shades of skin more attractive.

As the *Daily Mail* wrote in summarizing the study, "Women favor darker, brooding men... [they] pick men with darker complexions... because these are associated with sex, virility, mystery, villainy and danger."

Admit it: that bottle of Jergens is looking a little less ridiculous right about now, isn't it?

To see the effects of darker skin in action, let's re-examine our favorite humble-to-handsome transformation, shall we? Google Chris Pratt again, but this time ignore his eyebrows; instead, look at his skin tone.

What you'll find is that the handsome, leading-man version of Pratt has skin that's distinctly more tanned than his younger, still-relegated-to-comedic-relief self.

Now, it's possible that leading-man Pratt spends a lot more time in the sun than his goofily disheveled former self.

But if I were a betting man, I'd wager that Star-Lord's highly paid stylists have used self-tanning cream or something similar to help him achieve a darker, more attractive (and less acne-revealing) color.

Your Move:

Pick up some self-tanner and try it for yourself. Use it once a day, and if you're worried about accidentally going all Oompa Loompa, try cutting it with some regular sunscreen to dilute the color a bit.

9. Get Your Shirts (and the Rest of Your Shit) Tailored

The clothes don't make the man – but they can sure as hell make him look better.

Now that we've tackled the question of how to look more handsome from a grooming perspective, let's look at a few tweaks you can make to your wardrobe to improve your overall look.

By far the most effective thing you can do to upgrade your current wardrobe without buying anything new is get your shirts, pants and other core wardrobe pieces tailored.

Tailoring is the secret weapon of menswear. I'd much rather have a $100 suit that fit like a glove than a $10,000 suit that draped off my shoulders, bunched up at the ankles or otherwise didn't fit my frame.

And since good local tailors are easy to find thanks to review sites like Yelp and Google, this one should be a no-brainer.

Your Move(s):

Go through your closet and try on everything you own. Yep, everything.

Look in the mirror and ask yourself honestly if it fits as well as it could. If it doesn't look right, set it aside and start a pile of stuff you plan to have tailored.

Over the next week, start bringing in your clothes to have them altered. Bring in as many as you can at one time (while still leaving yourself something to wear, of course) and see if you can get a bulk discount from your tailor.

By the time you're done, you'll practically have a brand-new wardrobe that fits like a glove, for about a tenth of the price of what a brand new wardrobe would actually cost.

10. Tuck and Roll

Now that your shirt fits properly, it's time to learn how to wear it with style.

Tucking in your shirt – especially a shirt that's well cut – immediately makes you look more polished and put together. It conveys the message that you're conscientious and care about your appearance, both of which contribute to attractiveness.

Rolling up your sleeves, meanwhile, makes you look a little more relaxed, conveying that while you make an effort to look good, you're not too stuffy.

Your Move:

Tuck in your shirt and roll up your sleeves to simultaneously look more polished, more relaxed and more confident.

11. Wear a Tie – Even (and Especially) When You Don't Have To

Throwing a tie on with your (well-fitted) shirt instantly elevates the entire look.

Gone are the days when a man was expected to wear a suit and tie everywhere he went.

Outside of a few scarce professions and social functions, the standard for menswear today has never been more casual – which makes it easier than ever for you to handsomely stand out from the crowd. Because most guys today can barely be bothered to tuck their shirts in, something as simple as wearing a tie can instantly elevate you above your more casual peers.

In an article for *Forbes* about why you should dress 25 percent better than everyone else in the office, Carmine Gallo writes, "I asked a military hero the secret to leading a team into battle."

The military hero's reply?

"'That's a long answer... But I can tell you it all starts with how you're dressed the first time you meet them.

'If your pants are whiter, your shoes are shinier and your clothes are better pressed, you'll communicate confidence, a commanding presence. You're telegraphing that you're in charge.'"[37]

Fortunately, you don't need to wear the navy's dress whites to dress better than your peers – all you need is about ten bucks and an Amazon account.

Your Move:

Next time you're in a situation where a (well fitted and appropriately tucked) dress shirt would suffice, try throwing on a tie to elevate the look even further.

By dressing just slightly better than you have to, you'll gain handsome points in two ways.

First, you'll look even more put together and better dressed than the guy standing next to you.

Second, in so doing you'll instantly communicate that you're a cut above the norm, which will make you seem all the more attractive.

As I alluded to above, Amazon has literally thousands of options for ties ranging in price from two bucks to two hundred, so it should be easy to find one that fits both your budget and your tastes.

12. Blaze a New Trail

Here's how to elevate your look with one simple swap.

Not to be confused with its cousin the sport jacket, a blazer is basically a suit jacket with a more relaxed fit.

Because it has less structure in the shoulders, it gives off a more casual look and feel than a suit jacket, while still looking a hell of a lot sharper than a hoodie or sweatshirt.

The best part is that you can find these just about everywhere, from suit suppliers like J.Crew and Banana Republic to more casual stores like the Gap and even Old Navy.

Your Move:

Next time you're tempted to throw on a hoodie or a zip-up sweater, consider ditching them in favor of an unlined, unstructured blazer.

13. Shine Your Shoes

One of the best ways to out-dress the other guys is to make sure your look is on point all the way from head to toe.

The right pair of shoes (or boots) can elevate your look, but if you don't keep them in good shape, you'll miss out on their handsome benefits.

Remember what the military hero quoted above said? "If your pants are whiter, your shoes are shinier... you'll communicate confidence."

Your Move(s):

Pick up a shoe shining kit, which will have (pretty much) everything you need to restore the sheen to your shoes.

After a full week or two of wear, break out the shoe shine kit and give 'em a polish.

In between, keep an eye out for scuffs, mud or anything else that might make your shoes look less than ideal.

14. Convey Confidence with Your Body Language

Making sure your clothes and grooming are on point will go a long way toward making you look more handsome, but in order to really stand out you have to stand tall – or at least as tall as your frame can muster.

There are a lot of ways you can convey confidence, strength and attractiveness simply by using your body language effectively. But to keep it simple, just focus on the basics.

Generally speaking, men who stand up straight, occupy a lot of physical space by adopting a wide stance or spreading their arms, and move slowly and deliberately are considered more dominant, and thus more attractive.

As Harvard psychologist Amy Cuddy, author of the book *Presence*, has famously noted, adopting a powerful position with your body can actually make you feel more powerful.[38]

That effect extends to other people as well – carry yourself like a young George Clooney, and other people will (subconsciously) take notice.

Your Move:

Be more conscious of your body language. Stand with your feet shoulder width apart and keep your back straight, your chest out and your arms open (rather than crossed) to convey confidence.

CONCLUSION

"Self-confidence isn't something you're born with – it's something you build."

As I prepared to go into my boss's office I felt nervous, but excited.

This was about five years after the story I told you about in the introduction to this book, when I couldn't summon enough confidence to apply for a job I was qualified for.

I was now at a different company and working at a job I loved – one where the pay was good, my boss was encouraging and supportive, my colleagues were amazing and the work was interesting. While working for this company I had received promotions and raises, won industry awards for my work and truly believed I was in the perfect working environment.

And on this particular day, I was especially thrilled – because I was about to quit.

To most people (including my closest friends and family), leaving a job I just described as "the perfect working environment" probably didn't seem like a prudent, smart or particularly sound idea – especially since I didn't even have another job lined up.

But I was steadfast in my decision and excited about my future because, after years of building self-confidence, I had acquired a deep, unshakeable belief in myself and my abilities, and I knew that I was ready to make the leap.

The leap to what, you ask? To leaving the safe confines of a salaried position to go into business for myself. To working on my blog, IrreverentGent.com, full-time and sharing everything I've learned about building self-confidence with other guys who could stand to benefit from learning it. And, ultimately, to writing this book.

Just a few years earlier, I didn't have enough courage to even apply for a job that I was qualified for, and now I had built so much confidence that I felt ready to take a huge risk, to strike out on my own and to pursue a path that I previously could have only dreamed of.

In short, I had become a Man in Command of my own destiny.

And you can too.

After reading this book, you now have the tools you need to go from a shy, quiet and self-doubting guy to a strong, charming and self-confident man.

But a tool can't create anything unless a craftsman puts it to use. So don't wait another week, another day or even another minute to take control of your confidence.

Because as I told you way back in the introduction, self-confidence isn't something you're born with – it's something you build.

And it's time for you to start building yours.

NOTES

1. Stephen Covey. The 7 Habits of Highly Effective People (New York: Free Press, 1989), 98.
2. Nathaniel Branden. *The Six Pillars of Self-Esteem* (New York: Bantam, 1994), 4.
3. Nathaniel Branden. *The Six Pillars of Self-Esteem* (New York: Bantam, 1994), 26.
4. Darlene Lancer. "Low Self-Esteem is Learned." *Psych Central.* https://psychcentral.com/lib/low-self-esteem-is-learned/
5. Suzanne Lachmann. "10 Ways Low Self-Esteem Affects Women in Relationships." *Psychology Today.* https://www.psychologytoday.com/blog/me-we/201312/10-ways-low-self-esteem-affects-women-in-relationships
6. Darlene Lancer. "Low Self-Esteem is Learned." *Psych Central.* https://psychcentral.com/lib/low-self-esteem-is-learned/
7. "Confident People Get Promoted." *Healthy Living Magazine.* http://www.healthylivingmagazine.us/Articles/4895/

8. Nathaniel Branden. *The Six Pillars of Self-Esteem* (New York: Bantam, 1994), 11.
9. John Neffinger and Matthew Kohut. *Compelling People: The Hidden Qualities That Make Us Influential* (New York: Penguin, 2013), xi.
10. Meghan Casserly. "Top Five Personality Traits Employers Hire Most." *Forbes.* https://www.forbes.com/sites/meghancasserly/2012/10/04/top-five-personality-traits-employers-hire-most/
11. Hannah Furness. "Key to career success is confidence, not talent." *The Telegraph.* http://www.telegraph.co.uk/news/uknews/9474973/Key-to-career-success-is-confidence-not-talent.html
12. "Confident People Get Promoted." *Healthy Living Magazine.* http://www.healthylivingmagazine.us/Articles/4895/
13. Barbara L. Fredrickson, Michael A. Cohn, Kimberly A. Coffey, Jolynn Pek, and Sandra M. Finkel. "Open Hearts Build Lives: Positive Emotions, Induced Through Loving-Kindness Meditation, Build Consequential Personal Resources." *Journal of Personality and Social Psychology.* https://www.ncbi.nlm.nih.gov/pmc/articles/PMC3156028/
14. Heleen A Slagter, Antoine Lutz, Lawrence L Greischar, Andrew D Francis, Sander Nieuwenhuis, James M Davis, Richard J Davidson. "Mental Training Affects Distribution of Limited Brain Resources." *PLOS Biology.* http://journals.plos.org/plosbiology/article?id=10.1371/journal.pbio.0050138
15. Fadel Zeidana, Susan K. Johnson, Bruce J. Diamond, Zhanna David, Paula Goolkasian. "Mindfulness meditation improves cognition: evidence of brief mental training." *Science Direct.* http://www.sciencedirect.com/science/article/pii/S1053810010000681?via%3Dihub
16. The Greater Good Science Center. "Gratitude Defined."

University of California Berkeley. https://greatergood.berkeley.edu/gratitude/definition#why-practice
17. Seligman, M. P., Steen, T. A., Park, N., & Peterson, C. (2005). Positive Psychology Progress. *American Psychologist.* https://www.ncbi.nlm.nih.gov/pubmed/16045394
18. Negro M, Giardina S, Marzani B, Marzatico F. "Branched-chain amino acid supplementation does not enhance athletic performance but affects muscle recovery and the immune system." National Institutes of Health. https://www.ncbi.nlm.nih.gov/pubmed/18974721
19. Josh Axe. "Protein Foods: 8 Health Benefits of Foods High in Protein." https://draxe.com/protein-foods/
20. Kris Gunnars. "10 Reasons Why Sugar is Bad For You." *Health Line.* https://www.healthline.com/nutrition/10-disturbing-reasons-why-sugar-is-bad#section1
21. Alyson B. Goodman, Heidi M. Blanck, Bettylou Sherry, Sohyun Park, Linda Nebeling, Amy L. Yaroch. "Behaviors and Attitudes Associated With Low Drinking Water Intake Among US Adults, Food Attitudes and Behaviors Survey, 2007." *Preventing Chronic Disease.* https://www.cdc.gov/pcd/issues/2013/12_0248.htm
22. Tom Rath. *Eat Move Sleep: How Small Choices Lead to Big Changes* (Arlington: Mission Day, 2013), 13.
23. Tom Rath. *Eat Move Sleep: How Small Choices Lead to Big Changes* (Arlington: Mission Day, 2013), 16.
24. Susan Cain. "Are You Shy, Introverted, Both, or Neither (and Why Does It Matter)?" *Quiet Revolution.* https://www.quietrev.com/are-you-shy-introverted-both-or-neither-and-why-does-it-matter/
25. Susan Cain. *Quiet: The Power of Introverts in a World that Can't Stop Talking* (New York: Random House, 2012), 4.
26. Teresa Aubele and Susan Reynolds. "Happy Brain, Happy Life." *Psychology Today.* https://www.psychologytoday.com/blog/prime-your-gray-cells/201108/happy-brain-happy-life

27. Dale Carnegie. *How to Win Friends and Influence People* (New York: Simon & Schuster, 1936), 111.
28. Alyssa Detweiler. "9 Surprising Reasons Why You Should Smile More." *Inspyr.com.* https://inspiyr.com/9-benefits-of-smiling/
29. Sarah Stevenson. "There's Magic In Your Smile." *Psychology Today.* https://www.psychologytoday.com/blog/cutting-edge-leadership/201206/there-s-magic-in-your-smile
30. Charles Feng. "Looking Good: The Psychology and Biology of Beauty." *Journal of Young Investigators.* http://legacy.jyi.org/volumes/volume6/issue6/features/feng.html
31. Charles Feng. "Looking Good: The Psychology and Biology of Beauty." *Journal of Young Investigators.* http://legacy.jyi.org/volumes/volume6/issue6/features/feng.html
32. Nathaniel Branden. *The Six Pillars of Self-Esteem* (New York: Bantam, 1994).
33. B. J. W. Dixson, D. Sulikowski, A. Gouda-Vossos, M. J. Rantala, R. C. Brooks. "The masculinity paradox: facial masculinity and beardedness interact to determine women's ratings of men's facial attractiveness." *Journal of Evolutionary Biology.* http://dx.doi.org/10.1111/jeb.12958
34. Dana Oliver. "A Men's Eyebrow Grooming Guide In 6 Easy Steps." *HuffPost.* http://www.huffingtonpost.ca/entry/men-eyebrows-grooming_n_3749690
35. *GQ.* "What You Can Learn from the Most Opinionated Man in Fashion." https://www.gq.com/gallery/what-you-can-learn-from-michael-kors-february-2013#2
36. Andy Dolan. "Why men prefer fair-skinned maidens and women like dark, handsome strangers." *The Daily Mail.* http://www.dailymail.co.uk/sciencetech/article-535828/Why-men-prefer-fair-skinned-maidens-women-like-dark-handsome-strangers.html
37. Carmine Gallo. "Why You Should Dress 25% Better Than Everyone In The Office." *Forbes.* https://www.forbes.com/

sites/carminegallo/2016/08/27/why-you-should-dress-25-percent-better-than-everyone-in-the-office/#17eeff81409d

38. Amy Cuddy. *Presence: Bringing Your Boldest Self to Your Biggest Challenges* (New York: Little, Brown, 2015).

*Names have been changed to protect privacy.

ACKNOWLEDGMENTS

First and foremost, this book would not have been possible without the love and steadfast support of my family.

It was the encouragement and belief of my amazing wife Michelle that propelled me to start writing about my passion for self-improvement, and her patience and generosity of spirit that sustained me through the many days of doubt that I've encountered on this journey. This book, like all the best things I do, is for her.

My love of writing stems from a love of reading instilled in me early on by my parents, Bill and Loretta Bowden, whose home is constantly littered with books, newspapers and magazines. Thank you for not objecting too loudly when I declared that I wanted to spend your hard-earned money writing philosophical essays in undergrad; for encouraging me when I spent a little bit more learning how to refine my writing in journalism school; and for supporting me in those early days before I found my footing in the workforce. I owe the awards I've won, the skills I've cultivated and the career I've carved out for myself to your unwavering support for my writing.

In my family the love and support has always trickled downwards from the top, and at the top of our family tree sit my grandparents,

Angelo and Rina Longo. Your generosity, hard work and compassion have set an example for all of us. In addition, my grandpa has spent a lifetime being both the best dressed and the most charismatic guy in the room; I may have *written* the book on becoming confident and charming, but he inspired it.

And finally, my editor Michelle MacAleese of LifeTree Media helped me take what started as an expanded collection of blog posts and turn it into a complete and cohesive book. Both this book and its author benefited greatly from her experience and professionalism.

ABOUT THE AUTHOR

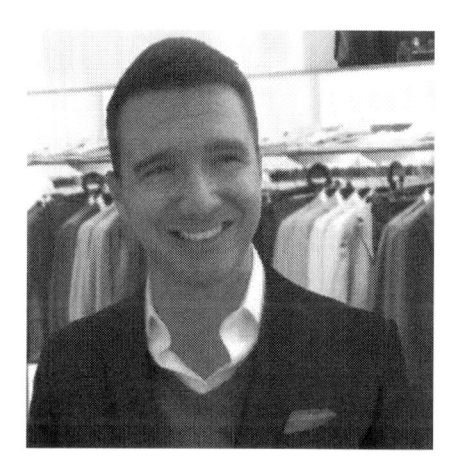

Dave Bowden is an award-winning blogger, writer and editor whose work has been featured in international magazines, national newspapers, and (most importantly) on his parents' fridge.

He founded IrreverentGent.com in 2015 to help guys overcome over-thinking, escape insecurity and take control of their confidence.

Connect with Dave online:
www.IrreverentGent.com
dave@irreverentgent.com